VOLUME ONE HUNDRED AND FIVE

ADVANCES IN PARASITOLOGY

Regional Network for Asian Schistosomiasis and Other Helminthic Zoonoses

VOLUME ONE HUNDRED AND FIVE

ADVANCES IN PARASITOLOGY

Regional Network for Asian Schistosomiasis and Other Helminthic Zoonoses

Edited by

XIAO-NONG ZHOU
National Institute of Parasitic Diseases, Chinese Center for Disease Control and Prevention; Chinese Center for Tropical Diseases Research; WHO Collaborating Centre for Tropical Diseases; National Center for International Research on Tropical Diseases; Key Laboratory of Parasite and Vector Biology, Ministry of Health, Shanghai, China

LYDIA LEONARDO
Institute of Biology, College of Science, University of the Philippines Diliman and University of the East Ramon Magsaysay Graduate School, Quezon City, The Philippines

ROBERT BERGQUIST
Geospatial Health, Ingerod, Brastad, Sweden

ELSEVIER

ACADEMIC PRESS
An imprint of Elsevier

Academic Press is an imprint of Elsevier
125 London Wall, London EC2Y 5AS, United Kingdom
The Boulevard, Langford Lane, Kidlington, Oxford OX5 1GB, United Kingdom
50 Hampshire Street, 5th Floor, Cambridge, MA 02139, United States
525 B Street, Suite 1650, San Diego, CA 92101, United States

First edition 2019

Notices
Knowledge and best practice in this field are constantly changing. As new research and experience broaden our understanding, changes in research methods, professional practices, or medical treatment may become necessary.

Practitioners and researchers must always rely on their own experience and knowledge in evaluating and using any information, methods, compounds, or experiments described herein. In using such information or methods they should be mindful of their own safety and the safety of others, including parties for whom they have a professional responsibility.

To the fullest extent of the law, neither the Publisher nor the authors, contributors, or editors, assume any liability for any injury and/or damage to persons or property as a matter of products liability, negligence or otherwise, or from any use or operation of any methods, products, instructions, or ideas contained in the material herein.

ISBN: 978-0-12-817718-1
ISSN: 0065-308X

For information on all Academic Press publications
visit our website at https://www.elsevier.com/books-and-journals

Publisher: Zoe Kruze
Acquisition Editor: Ashlie M. Jackman
Editorial Project Manager: Ana Claudia A. Garcia
Production Project Manager: Abdulla Sait
Cover Designer: Greg Harris

Typeset by SPi Global, India

Contents

Contributors ix
Preface: Sustained cooperation on research and control of neglected tropical diseases among multisectors and multipartners across borders in Southeast Asia xi

1. Milestones of networking and global engagements for the Regional Network on Asian Schistosomiasis and other Helminthic Zoonoses (RNAS$^+$) **1**
Lydia Leonardo, Robert Bergquist, Juerg Utzinger, Arve Lee Willingham, Remigio Olveda, and Xiao-Nong Zhou

1. Introduction 2
2. The preparatory stage 2
3. The first years of the network 3
4. Expansion: Creation of RNAS$^+$ 7
5. RNAS$^+$: Vision, mission, goals and strategies 8
6. Further expansion of RNAS$^+$ 9
7. Research projects: Objectives and outcomes 13
8. Global engagements: International stakeholders 18

References 20

2. Collaborative RNAS$^+$ research: Priorities and outcomes **23**
Lydia Leonardo, Robert Bergquist, Shi-Zhu Li, Shan Lv, Virak Khieu, Somphou Sayasone, Jing Xu, Remigio Olveda, Juerg Utzinger, and Xiao-Nong Zhou

1. Introduction 24
2. Epidemiological studies 24
3. Morbidity studies 29
4. Immunology and vaccine development 33
5. Diagnosis 35
6. Prevention and control 40

References 45
Further reading 51

3. Needs and coordination mechanism for capacity building by the RNAS+ **53**

Xiao-Nong Zhou, Lydia Leonardo, Juerg Utzinger, Shan Lv, Jing Xu, Arve Lee Willingham, Yan Lu, Don McManus, Shi-Zhu Li, Marilu Venturina, Remigio Olveda, and Robert Bergquist

1. Introduction 54
2. Need for capacity building 55
3. Improving capacity 57
4. Capacity building: Selected case studies 58
5. Capacity building opportunities 63
6. Conclusion 66

References 67

4. From country control programmes to translational research **69**

Lydia Leonardo, Robert Bergquist, Remigio Olveda, Fadjar Satrija, Banchob Sripa, Somphou Sayasone, Virak Khieu, Arve Lee Willingham, Juerg Utzinger, and Xiao-Nong Zhou

1. Introduction 70
2. Significant developments 71
3. Database for surveillance in the elimination phase 74
4. New guides for clinicians 78
5. High burdens of target diseases generate interest in control 80
6. Review of control programmes 82
7. Components needed for successful control programmes 84
8. Success stories: Elimination of LF 88
9. Conclusion 89

References 89

Further reading 92

5. Multi-disciplinary integration of networking through the RNAS+: Research on other target diseases **95**

Lydia Leonardo, Robert Bergquist, Shi-Zhu Li, Shan Lv, Virak Khieu, Somphou Sayasone, Jing Xu, Remigio Olveda, Juerg Utzinger, Banchob Sripa, Fadjar Satrija, Sirikachorn Tangkawattana, Helena Ullyartha, Khin Thet Wai, Hung Nguyen, and Xiao-Nong Zhou

1. Introduction 96
2. Neglected tropical diseases under the network 97

3. Food-borne trematodiases 98
4. Echinococcosis and cysticercosis 104
5. Lymphatic filariasis, soil-transmitted helminthiases and other helminthiases 105
References 108
Further reading 110

6. From inspiration to translation: Closing the gap between research and control of helminth zoonoses in Southeast Asia 111

Robert Bergquist, Lydia Leonardo, and Xiao-Nong Zhou

1. Introduction 112
2. Research activities and raison d'être 114
3. International research funding 117
4. What is still missing? 118
5. Lessons learnt and the way forward 119
References 121

7. Challenges and way forward 125

Lydia Leonardo, Robert Bergquist, Juerg Utzinger, Shi-Zhu Li, Marilu Venturina, and Xiao-Nong Zhou

1. Introduction 125
2. Way forward 130
References 132

Annex 1: Publications through RNAS⁺ platform *133*
Annex 2: The memory photos in the selected RNAS⁺ annual workshops *139*
Annex 3: Mapping the NTDs over RNAS⁺ countries *147*

Contributors

Robert Bergquist
Geospatial Health, Ingerod, Brastad, Sweden

Virak Khieu
National Helminth Control Program, National Center for Parasitology, Entomology and Malaria Control, Ministry of Health, Phnom Penh, Cambodia

Lydia Leonardo
Institute of Biology, College of Science, University of the Philippines Diliman and University of the East Ramon Magsaysay Graduate School, Quezon City, Philippines

Shi-Zhu Li
National Institute of Parasitic Diseases, Chinese Center for Disease Control and Prevention; Chinese Center for Tropical Diseases Research; WHO Collaborating Centre for Tropical Diseases; National Center for International Research on Tropical Diseases; Key Laboratory of Parasite and Vector Biology, Ministry of Health, Shanghai, China

Yan Lu
National Institute of Parasitic Diseases, Chinese Center for Disease Control and Prevention; Chinese Center for Tropical Diseases Research; WHO Collaborating Centre for Tropical Diseases; National Center for International Research on Tropical Diseases; Key Laboratory of Parasite and Vector Biology, Ministry of Health, Shanghai, China

Shan Lv
National Institute of Parasitic Diseases, Chinese Center for Disease Control and Prevention; Chinese Center for Tropical Diseases Research; WHO Collaborating Centre for Tropical Diseases; National Center for International Research on Tropical Diseases; Key Laboratory of Parasite and Vector Biology, Ministry of Health, Shanghai, China

Don McManus
QIMR Berghofer Medical Research Institute, Molecular Parasitology Laboratory, Brisbane, QLD, Australia

Hung Nguyen
Department of Parasitology, Institute of Ecology and Biological Resources, Vietnam Academy of Science and Technology, Hanoi, Vietnam

Remigio Olveda
Asian Tropical Foundation, Filinvest Corporate City, Research Institute for Tropical Medicine Compound, Muntinlupa, Philippines

Fadjar Satrija
Bogor Agricultural University (IPB), JL. Agatis, Kampus IPB, Bogor, Indonesia

Somphou Sayasone
Lao Tropical and Public Health Institute, Vientianne, Lao People's Democratic Republic

Banchob Sripa
Department of Pathology, Khon Kaen University, Khon Kaen, Thailand

Sirikachorn Tangkawattana
Department of Pathology, Khon Kaen University, Khon Kaen, Thailand

Helena Ullyartha
Ministry of Health, South Jakarta, Indonesia

Juerg Utzinger
Swiss Tropical and Public Health Institute, Basel, Switzerland

Marilu Venturina
Asian Tropical Foundation, Filinvest Corporate City, Research Institute for Tropical Medicine Compound, Muntinlupa, Philippines

Khin Thet Wai
Department of Medical Research, Ministry of Health & Sports, Yangon, Myanmar

Arve Lee Willingham
One Health Center for Zoonoses and Tropical Veterinary Medicine, Ross University School of Veterinary Medicine, Basseterre, St. Kitts, West Indies

Jing Xu
National Institute of Parasitic Diseases, Chinese Center for Disease Control and Prevention; Chinese Center for Tropical Diseases Research; WHO Collaborating Centre for Tropical Diseases; National Center for International Research on Tropical Diseases; Key Laboratory of Parasite and Vector Biology, Ministry of Health, Shanghai, China

Xiao-Nong Zhou
National Institute of Parasitic Diseases, Chinese Center for Disease Control and Prevention; Chinese Center for Tropical Diseases Research; WHO Collaborating Centre for Tropical Diseases; National Center for International Research on Tropical Diseases; Key Laboratory of Parasite and Vector Biology, Ministry of Health, Shanghai, China

Preface: Sustained cooperation on research and control of neglected tropical diseases among multisectors and multipartners across borders in Southeast Asia

Abstract

This special issue is going to introduce the origins of the "Regional Network on Asian Schistosomiasis (RNAS)" which can be traced back to 1996. RNAS was originally a collaboration of scientists from China and Philippines, and then expanded to Cambodia, Indonesia, Japan and Laos, with focusing on research and control of schistosomiasis japonica. However, at its fifth meeting in Bali, Indonesia in 2005, more countries such as Vietnam, Thailand and Korea were brought on board along with a string of neglected tropical diseases such as cysticercosis, clonorchiasis, opisthorchiasis and fascioliasis, and RNAS thus became RNAS$^+$. We all expected that the progress made so far will be enough to persuade donors to assist RNAS$^+$ in its current activities and forward movement.

The origins of the "Regional Network on Asian Schistosomiasis (RNAS)" can be traced back to a discussion during a 1996 workshop in Nanjing, China. This meeting, "Research, Surveillance and Control of Schistosomiasis Japonica", sponsored by the UNICEF/UNDP/World Bank/WHO Special Programme for Research and Training in Tropical Diseases (TDR) initiated the idea of a network taking the shape of a bid to coral stakeholders to step up the fight against schistosomiasis japonica in Southeast Asia.

Research on schistosomiasis has a long tradition in China and the Philippines, the two countries in the region with the largest burdens of the disease. Operational research has always been an important component of their national control programmes which have both contributed to past successes in reducing the impact of schistosomiasis. The 1980s saw the beginning of a multidisciplinary approach made possible with input from TDR, the Rockefeller Foundation and the creation of Tropical Medicine Research Centers (TMRC) with grants from the US National Institutes of Health. This fostered strong collaboration between national research institutes and research groups within and outside the region including countries as far away as Australia, UK and USA. The role played by the World Bank is particularly pivotal by focusing activities on control which initially led to a dramatic drop in prevalence of the disease in both countries, but the final outcome was different in China and the Philippines. While the Bank initiated work in the Philippines already in the 1980s fully concentrating on supporting the control programme, about 3% of the 10-year total World Bank Loan Project (WBLP) in China (1991–2000) was set aside for research. It should be added that the WBLP, including matching funds from the Chinese Government, amounted to more than 80 million US dollars and, at the time, constituted the biggest project undertaken for any parasitic disease. Importantly, research benefitted handsomely and produced breakthroughs in many areas resulting in testing of new strategies, progress on vaccine and drug development and initiation of the use of Geographical Information Systems (GIS). While the time after the World Bank input, prevalence surveys have become irregular in the Philippines and mostly limited to highly endemic areas, China has been able to sustain a country-wide control programme and largely kept prevalence from rising. Naturally, the current improvements in the Chinese economy are an important factor, but the role played by WBLP research component should not be underestimated.

RNAS was originally a collaboration of scientists from Cambodia, China, Indonesia, Japan, Laos and the Philippines exclusively focused on research, surveillance and control of schistosomiasis japonica. However, at its fifth meeting in Bali, Indonesia in 2005 the number of participants had grown substantially and a strong need was felt to also do something for the other neglected diseases in the region. The network had chalked up an impressive number of accomplishments and started to make a sustained impact on the research and control of schistosomiasis. The challenges were discussed with a view to find the best possible future direction. The knowledge that the network was widely seen as a model for other initiatives encouraged the view that the RNAS vision should expand and accommodate other neglected parasitic diseases and new member countries. Henceforth, Vietnam, Thailand and Korea were brought onboard along with a string of endemic diseases such as cysticercosis, clonorchiasis, opisthorchiasis and fascioliasis, and RNAS thus became RNAS^{+}.

The progress and new developments were clearly at hand in the follow-up meeting in the historic city of Lijiang, China in 2007, which attracted 150 participants from 19 countries and international organizations. The form of this meeting was an open forum exchanging information on the various diseases in the different countries and regions with the aim of sharing documentation and conclusions with regional Ministries of Health to enable more effective research, treatment and disease control. RNAS+ is now at an important juncture. It is faced with a situation where we have the means to control many of the different target diseases, but this asks for immediate, strong action, both with regard to research and control. The ideas, along which we have been working over the last decade, have shown that progress can be made with a relatively small network and limited funding. However, the stakes have increased and the larger vision demands improved financial support to permit a continuous exchange of ideas and data to make it possible for national researchers and control managers to work together and be in contact with international scientists on a daily basis. This goal is being achieved thanks to modern computers and continuous Internet access. It is hoped that the progress made so far, evidenced by the papers presented here, will be enough to persuade donors to assist RNAS+ in its current activities and forward movement.

For more information on The Regional Network for Research, Surveillance and Control for Asian Schistosomiasis (RNAS) access rnas.ipd.org.cn

Xiao-Nong Zhou
National Institute of Parasitic Diseases, Chinese Center for Disease Control and Prevention, Shanghai, China
Chinese Center for Tropical Diseases Research, Shanghai, China
WHO Collaborating Centre for Tropical Diseases, Shanghai, China
National Center for International Research on Tropical Diseases, Shanghai, China
Key Laboratory of Parasite and Vector Biology, Ministry of Health, Shanghai, China
Lydia Leonardo
Institute of Biology, College of Science, University of the Philippines Diliman and University of the East Ramon Magsaysay Graduate School, Quezon City, The Philippines
Robert Bergquist
Geospatial Health, Ingerod, Brastad, Sweden

CHAPTER ONE

Milestones of networking and global engagements for the Regional Network on Asian Schistosomiasis and other Helminthic Zoonoses (RNAS$^+$)

Lydia Leonardo[a,*], Robert Bergquist[b], Juerg Utzinger[c], Arve Lee Willingham[d], Remigio Olveda[e], Xiao-Nong Zhou[f,g,h,i,j]

[a]Institute of Biology, College of Science, University of the Philippines Diliman and University of the East Ramon Magsaysay Graduate School, Quezon City, Philippines
[b]Geospatial Health, Ingerod, Brastad, Sweden
[c]Swiss Tropical and Public Health Institute, Basel, Switzerland
[d]One Health Center for Zoonoses and Tropical Veterinary Medicine, Ross University School of Veterinary Medicine, Basseterre, St. Kitts, West Indies
[e]Asian Tropical Foundation, Filinvest Corporate City, Research Institute for Tropical Medicine Compound, Muntinlupa, Philippines
[f]National Institute of Parasitic Diseases, Chinese Center for Disease Control and Prevention, Beijing, China
[g]Chinese Center for Tropical Diseases Research, Shanghai, China
[h]WHO Collaborating Centre for Tropical Diseases, Shanghai, China
[i]National Center for International Research on Tropical Diseases, Shanghai, China
[j]Key Laboratory of Parasite and Vector Biology, Ministry of Health, Shanghai, China
*Corresponding author: e-mail address: lydialeonardo1152@gmail.com

Contents

1. Introduction 2
2. The preparatory stage 2
3. The first years of the network 3
4. Expansion: Creation of RNAS$^+$ 7
5. RNAS$^+$: Vision, mission, goals and strategies 8
6. Further expansion of RNAS$^+$ 9
7. Research projects: Objectives and outcomes 13
   7.1 Three projects funded by TDR 13
   7.2 First project funded by the International Development Research Centre in Canada (IDRC) 14
   7.3 Control and elimination of helminth zoonoses in the Greater Mekong Subregion 17
8. Global engagements: International stakeholders 18
References 20

Advances in Parasitology, Volume 105
ISSN 0065-308X
https://doi.org/10.1016/bs.apar.2019.07.006

Abstract

This paper introduces the three stages of development of the Regional Network on Asian Schistosomiasis and other Helminthic Zoonoses (RNAS$^+$), namely the preparatory stage, the strengthening stage and the expanding stage. Significant achievements have been made through the help of RNAS$^+$, particularly on research on helminthiases. As scientists, researchers, academics work closer with control authorities, elimination of these diseases is slowly getting nearer and within reach. RNAS$^+$, at present can boast of the following strengths: (i) strong collaboration in the regional research area with support from experts on research and control; (ii) presence of experts in various areas who can improve and promote both research and control; (iii) RNAS$^+$ has been successful in translating research output to field application; (iv) setting up a platform that is capable of advancing the mechanisms of sharing information through its website, databases, publications and meetings; (v) RNAS$^+$ has proved that it is capable of undertaking joint collaborative projects on operational research through multi-country, multi-disease using multi-disciplinary approach and involving different academic and research institutions in the region. Most importantly, experts who are members of RNAS$^+$ are also linked with control programmes of the endemic member countries in the region.

1. Introduction

The history of the Regional Network on Asian Schistosomiasis (RNAS) can be traced back to 1996 during an international meeting in Nanjing, PR China. Since then, significant achievements on research and control of helminths have been made that inspired developing countries to aspire beyond control and prevention of schistosomiasis which is elimination. The development of RNAS and RNAS$^+$ has attracted much attention in the international community as the network transitioned through the following three development stages and emerging as the longest surviving network of this nature.

2. The preparatory stage

The Regional Network on Asian Schistosomiasis (RNAS) originated out of a discussion at an international workshop held in Nanjing, PR China in 1996. This meeting, 'Research, Surveillance and Control of Asian Schistosomiasis' was supported by the UNICEF/UNDP/World Bank/WHO Special Programme for Research and Training in Tropical Diseases (TDR). Two years later, on September 8–10, 1998, 70 scientists and representatives from control authorities from the People's Republic of

China (PR China), the Philippines and other countries gathered in the Chinese city of Wuxi to plan for a network based on intersectoral, interregional and international collaboration for research, surveillance and control of schistosomiasis japonica. The proceedings produced after this meeting published by McGarvey et al. (1999) marked the informal beginning of the Regional Network on Asian Schistosomiasis (RNAS) that was formally established in the year 2000 as an initiative to bring together all possible stakeholders in a bid to step up the fight against schistosomiasis japonica.

3. The first years of the network

The first meeting of the newly founded network was held on February 18–19, 2000 in Tagaytay City, the Philippines and attended by 28 participants from Australia, China, Denmark, Japan, Switzerland and the Philippines. The meeting formally organized the overall plan to control schistosomiasis japonica in all endemic areas in Southeast Asia (Zhou et al., 2002). A total of 15 papers covering progress on research and control of Asian schistosomiasis were presented and a round table discussion was conducted to draw up the next 2-year plan of work of the new organization. One and a half years later, on the first 2 days of July 2001, the network returned to Wuxi, PR China for its second official meeting which drew 38 participants representing government health agencies, research institutes on human and animal parasites and the academe from Australia, China, Denmark, Japan, Philippines and USA and for the first time, also from Indonesia. Representatives from TDR and the Western Pacific Regional Office (WPRO) of the World Health Organization (WHO) were also present. Reports presented included updates on diagnostic techniques, immunological studies. For the first time, a major session was devoted to the use of geographical information systems (GIS) for monitoring transmission and various issues related to control of schistosomiasis.

Two additional meetings, 3–4 (Table 1) followed, the first in Cambodia and the next in Lao PDR. The third meeting attracted 73 participants representing 12 countries and international organizations. Participants gathered in historic Phnom Penh for the latest updates given by scientists from Australia, China, Denmark, Germany, Indonesia, Japan, Laos, Sweden, the Philippines and USA. The network chair, Dr. Feng Zheng of the National Institute of Parasitic Diseases (NIPD) in Shanghai, PR China, made a strong call to consider capability strengthening aspects as part of the activities and thus create a strengthened RNAS, tentatively called SRNAS.

Table 1 Overview of meeting activities within the RNAS/RNAS$^+$ framework.

Meeting place	No.	Time	Focus of training course	Outcome
Nanjing, PR China	–	1996		Conclusion to initiate network
Wuxi, PR China	–	September 8–10, 1998		Preparatory discussions
Tagaytay City, Philippines	1	February 18–19, 2000		Formal organization of the 'Regional Network on Asian Schistosomiasis' (RNAS)
Wuxi, PR China	2	July 1–2, 2001		
Phnom Penh, Cambodia	3			Inclusion of Cambodia as RNAS member approved
Vientiane, Lao PDR	4	November 25–27, 2003		Inclusion of Lao PDR as RNAS member approved. TDR beginning to fund research specific network projects
Bali, Indonesia	5	August 8–10, 2005	Research Ethics	Expansion into other diseases (cysticercosis, clonorchiasis, opisthorchiasis, paragonimiasis and fascioliasis) and countries (Vietnam, Thailand, South Korea and Japan) changing into 'Regional Network on Asian Schistosomiasis and other Helminthic Zoonoses' (RNAS$^+$)

Muntinlupa, Philippines	6	September 11–15, 2006	GIS in epidemiology and surveillance of parasitic diseases conducted in Bohol in central Philippines.	
Lijiang, PR China	7	September 5–6, 2007	Burden Assessment of Important Helminth Zoonoses	RNAS$^+$ registered as a non-government, non-profit organization with the Philippine Securities and Exchange Commission effective August 31, 2017.
Jeju, South Korea	8	October 1–2, 2008		Meeting together with the scientific sessions on schistosomiasis at the 17th meeting of ICTMM
Vientiane, Lao PDR	9	October 19–20, 2009		RNAS$^+$ vision marked as fully compatible with WPRO's research strategic plan
Wuxi, PR China	10	November 16–19, 2010	Climate change and dynamic transmission modelling	Regional Research Plan of Action for Infectious Diseases of Poverty presented
Siem Reap, Cambodia	11	October 17–19, 2011	Social Marketing	Inclusion of Vietnam as RNAS$^+$ member approved
Hanoi, Vietnam	12	November 8–9, 2012	Serology and Molecular Techniques in Diagnosis of Parasitic Infections and Their Vectors	Focus on NTDs; opening of Facebook account
Khon Kaen, Thailand	13	October 24–26, 2013	Geospatial techniques for Public Health	Inclusion of Myanmar as RNAS$^+$ member approved

Continued

Table 1 Overview of meeting activities within the RNAS/RNAS$^+$ framework.—cont'd

Meeting place	No.	Time	Focus of training course	Outcome
Bogor, Indonesia	14	October 13–14, 2014	Conventional and Molecular Techniques for Helminthiasis Diagnosis	Preliminary report on suspected schistosomiasis in Myanmar presented
Philippines	15	July 23–24, 2015	Use of LAMP and Miracidial Hatching as Diagnostic Tools in Schistosomiasis	A donor meeting was held with several presentations
Yangon, Myanmar	16	October 27–28, 2016		Memorandum of understanding signed with African countries to strengthen schistosomiasis research
Vientiane, Lao PDR	17	October 24–25, 2017		
Shanghai, PR China	18	June 25–26, 2018		Inclusion of Malaysia as RNAS$^+$ member approved, meeting together with the 'Fourth Symposium on Surveillance Response Systems for Tropical Diseases Elimination'

The fourth meeting was held in 2003 in Vientiane, Lao PDR on November 25–27, showing the largest number of delegates so far, which also included industry, e.g., Shin Pong, the first producer of praziquantel besides Merck AG in Germany. After the two-day presentation of progress reports, country reports, research results and round table discussions, participants expressed strong support for the continuous exchange of experts among the member countries. Now with an established record of participation in scientific assemblies, the network started addressing problems, such as the urgency to increase awareness about ethical issues, the need to establish guidelines for surveillance and the standardization of a training manual for use in endemic areas. Annual reporting of data from the member countries was also encouraged together with efforts to elucidate the morbidity index for schistosomiasis. Participants also expressed commitment to assist the Ministry or Department of Health of member countries. Discussions of how to absorb training and capability strengthening into the network continued.

These years marked the transition to SRNAS and this stronger RNAS featured stronger communications among members through the creation of an internet homepage that enabled continued exchange of information on diagnosis, surveillance and control of schistosomiasis. As the organization made its way into its fourth year of existence, the benefits of membership had become clear and obvious. Participants agreed that the meetings had indeed become a useful vehicle for in-depth discussion and dissemination of new information. Outcomes of researches and results of new control modalities continued to fan optimism in possibly eliminating schistosomiasis. Multi-country research projects on different aspects of the disease achieved widespread sustainable collaboration among scientists from all the member countries. At this time TDR also began funding research projects from the network.

4. Expansion: Creation of RNAS+

The fifth meeting of the network took place in Bali, Indonesia on August 8–10, 2005. This became an occasion for the members to take a long hard look at the 6 years of the existence of their organization. It was attended by 60 participants from the Asian member countries as well as representatives of industry, this time Lonza Ltd., the Swiss provider of Bayluscide, as well as other international partners (Denmark, Sweden and Switzerland) together with representatives from TDR, WHO and WPRO. In addition to the usual presentations and updates in the field of schistosomiasis, the members also reviewed the organization's past progress taking note of achievements and accomplishments and its impact on the region. The task of confronting the challenges and the problems faced by RNAS was discussed with a view to track the best possible direction for the organization. Encouraged by the knowledge that the network has served as a model for other initiatives like the one contemplated for the same disease in Africa and an impetus for groups working on other helminth diseases, the participants responded to the call for change. The decision was to expand the vision and eventually reconfigure the network to accommodate new diseases and new member countries. Henceforth, the network expanded its target from schistosomiasis to a spectrum of other parasitic diseases such as cysticercosis, clonorchiasis, opisthorchiasis, paragonimiasis and fascioliasis with the corollary task of encouraging other endemic countries, such as Japan, South Korea, Thailand and Vietnam and to become RNAS members.

In its expanded form, the network was renamed Regional Network on Asian Schistosomiasis and other Helminthic Zoonoses (RNAS$^+$) with the larger vision of becoming the recognized platform for evidence-based information and intersectoral communication bridging the gap between research scientists and control authorities for the prevention of neglected tropical diseases in Southeast Asia. Its mission is to provide a forum for the exchange and dissemination of information about current researches and developments on prevention and control of Asian schistosomiasis and targeted, neglected tropical parasitic diseases including clonorchiasis, cysticercosis, fascioliasis, opisthorchiasis and paragonimiasis through intersectoral collaboration and communication among scientists and control authorities. As a result, more than 90% of all research institutions and control authorities in the nine member countries working on the RNAS$^+$ target diseases are represented in the network.

5. RNAS$^+$: Vision, mission, goals and strategies

RNAS$^+$ by now has become a force in multidisciplinary research and multisectoral collaboration among professionals, scientists and public health experts. In its first 10 years, the network passed through three stages of development. In the establishment stage, from 1999 to 2001, three regular scientific meetings were held and information sharing and collaboration between the Chinese and Filipino scientists expanded noticeably. There were further suggestions to include other members such as Laos and Cambodia which are endemic for schistosomiasis mekongi and Japan which was endemic for schistosomiasis japonica in the past but able to eliminate the disease in the 1990s. Indonesia which has three focal endemic schistosomiasis areas in the island of Sulawesi already attended the 2001 meeting in Wuxi. From a technical point of view, the importance of GIS and remote-sensing as a tool to monitor schistosomiasis had already been recognized at this time. In fact, remote-sensing was in fact first used for schistosomiasis in the Philippines (Cross et al., 1984).

From 2002 to 2004, in the second or strengthening stage, communications were further strengthened by the creation of the network's internet homepage enabling continuous exchange of information and data on the diagnosis, surveillance and control of *Schistosoma japonicum*. Research and training standardized methods in surveys of areas endemic for schistosomiasis. Research grants were awarded by TDR for three projects, i.e. application of immunodiagnostic kits, standardization of an ultrasound protocol, and development of survey tools for animal schistosomiasis. These grants encouraged the expansion of the network through participation of four countries endemic for oriental schistosomiasis in surveys of schistosomiasis japonica and mekongi in animals and humans.

The third stage, the phase of expansion, started in 2005 when the network expanded its targeted diseases to other helminth zoonoses such as cysticercosis, clonorchiasis, fascioliasis, opisthorchiasis, and paragonimiasis inviting countries endemic for these additional diseases, such as Japan, South Korea, Thailand and Vietnam. The possible coordination and collaboration with the other networks, such as the Regional Network on Schistosomiasis in Africa (RNSA) were raised in the 2005 meeting in Bali, Indonesia. The RNAS$^+$ structure was also formalized especially strengthening the secretariat of the network to facilitate communication. The chair of the network was given a term of 2 years after which the elected vice chair would take over. The need for the network to be registered as an official organization was also raised.

6. Further expansion of RNAS$^+$

The now expanded RNAS$^+$ met in the Philippines on September 11–15, 2006 which marked the 100th year of discovery of *S. japonicum* in the Philippines. Updates on other helminth zoonoses (cysticercosis, clonorchiasis, fascioliasis, opisthorchiasis and paragonimiasis) in the region were provided for the first time aside from the regular status reports on schistosomiasis from the endemic member countries. The organization also saw the need to formalize the governance of RNAS$^+$. Additional objectives such as disease mapping, training and advocacy were added to the original objectives of the network on research, control and surveillance of schistosomiasis. A training course on the application of GIS in epidemiology and surveillance of parasitic diseases was also conducted in the resort island of Bohol in central Philippines.

The seventh meeting of the network in Lijiang, China in 2007 attracted a total of 150 participants from 19 countries and international organizations. Since the venue was in China, the largest contingent of attendees (51%) were from the PR China. The conference was supported in part by the Chinese Ministry of Health in, TDR, the Danish Bilharziasis Laboratory (DBL) and the Global Network on Geospatial Health (GnosisGIS).

By this year, the network has been successfully registered as a non-governmental and non-profit organization with the Philippine Securities and Exchange Commission effective August 31, 2017. The officers of the network included Dr. Remigio Olveda from the Philippines as president; Dr. Zhou Xiaonong from PR China as vice president; Dr. Lydia Leonardo from the Philippines as secretary and Ms. Marilou Venturina from the Philippines as treasurer. For the first time, a representative from RNSA (Regional Network on Schistosomiasis in Africa) attended the meeting giving a report on the African network.

The eighth meeting of the network was held in Jeju, South Korea and incorporated as scientific sessions on schistosomiasis at the 17th International Congress for Tropical Medicine and Malaria between September 30 and October 2, 2008. Seven scientific sessions were organized by the network in the international congress that included international network for control; current status of vaccine programme; genomics and proteomics; disease burden; epidemiology; new tools for prophylaxis and treatment and clinical epidemiology.

The ninth meeting of RNAS$^+$ in Vientiane, Lao PDR on October 19–20, 2009 confirmed how the vision of RNAS$^+$ is fully compatible with WPRO's research strategic plan as well as with TDR's global vision. The ninth meeting eventually became a forum to refine and update WPRO's Research Strategic Plan Draft; to identify issues and operational research priorities that address key programmatic gaps in research areas of RNAS$^+$'s target diseases; and to reassess the roles of RNAS$^+$, define its strategies and future plans in contributing to the development of the NTD research agenda in Asia.

The network celebrated its 10th anniversary on November 16–19, 2010 back in Wuxi at the Jiangsu Institute of Parasitic Diseases (JIPD) where it was first conceptualized in 1998. A representative of RNSA talked about how the African network has influenced national and regional decision on schistosomiasis research and control. The Regional Research Plan of Action for Infectious Diseases of Poverty was presented by Dr. Jun Nakagawa of Western Pacific Regional Office of the WHO. The importance of networks and south to south collaborations was reiterated by Dr. Glenn Laverach, a leader in health promotion, public health and empowerment who worked for more than 30 years in Europe, Asia, Africa and the Pacific region. A training course on climate change and dynamic transmission modelling was attended by junior scientists.

The inclusion of Vietnam in the board of RNAS$^+$ was approved on the 11th meeting of the network October 17–19, 2011 at Siem Reap in Cambodia. The need for social marketing of RNAS$^+$ was also noted in the business meeting. The 12th meeting held for the first time in Hanoi, Vietnam was marked by presentation of member countries of diseases other than those targeted by RNAS$^+$, particularly neglected tropical diseases such as STH, filariasis, food-borne trematode diseases and others like trichinosis and angiostrongylosis. The network also decided to create a Facebook account for RNAS$^+$ in addition to the homepage to augment communication and visibility of the network.

The 13th meeting held for the first time in Thailand on October 24–26, 2013 marked the nomination and acceptance of Myanmar as a member country of RNAS$^+$. The plan to participate in the EcoHealth Conference in Montreal, Canada in August 2014 was approved which allowed RNAS$^+$ members to present their results on the multi-country, multi-disciplinary IDRC project. The meeting was capped by a visit to Thailand's trans-disciplinary Eco-Health project called the Lawa Model (Sripa et al., 2017). A half-day training on geospatial techniques for public health purposes was also given at this time.

The 14th meeting that took place in Bogor, Indonesia on October 13–14, 2014 was held simultaneously with two other international meetings, namely the fifth Annual Meeting of the Southeast Asian Veterinary Schools Association and the third Scientific Meeting of the Indonesian Veterinary Schools Association. A representative from Myanmar participated for the first time in the meeting giving a preliminary report on suspected schistosomiasis and other NTDs in this country.

At the 15th meeting, held in the Philippines for the third time in 2015, the RNAS$^+$ board decided to keep the website in China but set up an additional platform for communication with member countries and other people who could be interested to join the webpage. Dr. Shan Lu, NIPD, PR

China reported that a memorandum of understanding has been made between PR China and eight African countries to initiate South/South collaboration on schistosomiasis. A pilot study on schistosomiasis would be conducted in Tanzania. The board approved the inclusion of Dr. Mario Jiz from the Philippines as replacement of Dr. Luz Acosta who had migrated to Canada. A donors' meeting was also held where several presentations were made.

October 27–28, 2016 saw the 16th meeting of RNAS$^+$ for the first time in Myanmar. Replacements for retiring members of the board were approved such as those for Dr. Muth Sinuon in the person of Dr. Virak Khieu from Cambodia and Dr. Khay for Dr. Khin from Myanmar. A memorandum of understanding was signed with African countries to strengthen collaboration and research on schistosomiasis there. A move to organize an e-mail group was proposed for the purpose of sustaining discussion even beyond the regular annual meeting of the network. Issues, such as surveillance, criteria for elimination and the different phases of control, problems with mass drug administration (MDA) need for more sensitive diagnostics, development of new control strategies and challenges presently faced by member countries were addressed.

The 17th meeting of the network was held for the third time in Lao PDR in Vientiane October 24–25, 2017. The assumption of Dr. Somphou Sayasone of the RNAS$^+$ presidency was announced. There was an intense discussion on the development of sensitive diagnostic tests especially in the light of the progress achieved by member countries in controlling RNAS$^+$ target endemic diseases. Preliminary reports were presented on the results of the consultative meeting to accelerate elimination of Asian schistosomiasis held in May 2017 in Shanghai. The network decided however to await official results of the consultative meeting before developing any framework on schistosomiasis elimination. The same decision was made to base guidelines for cut-off for MDA (20% vs. 10%) on the results of the expert consultation on Food-Borne trematodiases (FBTs). It was decided to produce a book about RNAS$^+$ for the occasion of the 20th anniversary celebration of its founding.

The 18th meeting of RNAS$^+$ was held in Shanghai, PR China (the fifth time in PR China) on June 25–26, 2018 embedded as special sessions in the Fourth Symposium on Surveillance Response Systems for Tropical Disease Elimination. Dr. Somphou Sayasone from Lao PDR assumed the presidency of RNAS$^+$ for a term of 2 years from 2018 to 2020 and Dr. Virak Khieu from Cambodia was elected vice president. Malaysia was accepted as the 11th member country of the network with Dr. Vickneshwaran Muthu, senior principal assistant director from Zoonoses Sector, Disease Control Division, Ministry of Health in Malaysia as member of the RNAS+ board. The board recognized the significant contribution of Malaysia in the field of NTDs particularly in the development of diagnostic tests for lymphatic filariasis.

7. Research projects: Objectives and outcomes

7.1 Three projects funded by TDR

In 2002, during the second meeting of RNAS in PR China, Dr. Steve Wayling, TDR informed the network that funds, as well as opportunities for research support, were open to member countries as well as individuals. At the third meeting of the network held in Phnom Penh, Cambodia in 2003, three round table discussions were conducted to flesh out the details of three research subprojects to be submitted by the network for funding from WHO TDR. These subprojects were 'Application and evaluation of the dipstick dye immunoassay kit for community diagnosis of schistosomiasis mekongi in Cambodia and Lao PDR' coordinated by Dr. Zhu Yinchang, Director of the Jiangsu Institute of Parasitic Diseases of China; 'Standardization of ultrasound findings in Asian Schistosomiasis' coordinated by Dr. Remigio Olveda of the Research Institute for Tropical Medicine (RITM), Muntinlupa, the Philippines and 'Asian Schistosomiasis in animal hosts' coordinated by Dr. Lin Jiaojiao of the Institute of Animal Husbandry of Shanghai, PR China. Eventually, research grants were awarded by TDR for three projects.: application of immunodiagnostic kits; standardization of the ultrasonography; and development of survey tools for animal schistosomiasis.

The previous year, 2002, Dr. Zhu of JIPD, PR China, had informed the network on the development of this rapid diagnostic tool in their laboratory. The technique which is similar to ELISA uses schistosome egg antigens (SEA) conjugated with a colloidal dye to detect the presence of antibodies against SEA in the serum. The sensitivity of the test ranges from 94.1% to 96.7% and specificity is from 96.7% to 100% (Zhu et al., 2002). This Dipstick Dye Immunoassay (DDIA) takes 5–10 min to complete, is simple to prepare, does not require special equipment and the dye-conjugated antigen is stable at room temperature for 6 months. To evaluate the usefulness of the DDIA kit in the diagnosis of schistosomiasis mekongi, the project was carried out in Lao PDR and Cambodia training nine professionals from the National Center for Parasitology of Cambodia.

In Cambodia, the sensitivity was recorded at 97.1%, correctly diagnosing 33 out of 34 infected people, while in Lao PDR, a sensitivity of 98.6% (69/70) was noted. None of 114 residents living in a non-endemic area in Cambodia tested positive. However, a 18.3% cross-reaction with *Opisthorchis viverrini* was found. The results support the notion that the DDIA using *S. japonicum* SEA antigens can safely be implemented for the diagnosis of schistosomiasis mekongi, but false positive results in areas could appear in areas co-endemic for *O. viverrini* (Zhu et al., 2005).

For the second project, Dr. Christoph Hatz of the Swiss Tropical Institute (TPI) in Basel, Switzerland (now Swiss TIPH) and local collaborators presented ultrasound findings of morbidity due to *S. japonicum* and *S. mekongi.* With regards to network findings, there are distinctive signs in *S. japonicum* compared to none for *S. mekongi.* Results were compared to previous efforts to standardize the use of ultrasound in schistosomiasis made in Egypt (Cairo Working Group, 1992) and Niamey, Niger (TDR, 1996). For Asian schistosomiasis, similar discussions had been carried out in meetings in Hunan in 1992, Leyte in 1997, Wuhan in 2000, Yueyang in 2001 and Phnom Penh in 2002. (Leonardo and Bergquist, 2002; Zhou et al., 2002, 2010). Dr. Hatz stressed the need for standardizing the image patterns. For example, according to A (normal); B (questionable); C and D (different degrees of periportal fibrosis; E (strong reticular network of the liver; and E and F (observation of wide meshes indicating serious morbidity). He also presented potential confounders in the assessment of lesions due to *S. japonicum* such as liver cirrhosis, fatty liver, chronic hepatitis, liver tumours and other reasons for portal hypertension. For this project, a workshop was conducted in Hunan, PR China entitled 'Standardization of ultrasonography in schistosomiasis', and a report was drafted and eventually published (Li et al., 2004).

For the project on schistosomiasis in animals, a workshop on diagnostic tests was held at the DBL (Danish Bilharzhiasis Laboratory) in Denmark in September 2003 attended by 16 participants from eight countries including Cambodia, China, Indonesia, Lao PDR and the Philippines. The purpose of the workshop was to demonstrate, compare and reach consensus about diagnostic tests to be used for surveys, control and surveillance on animal schistosomiasis in Asia (Olveda et al., 2010; Zhou et al., 2008).

7.2 First project funded by the International Development Research Centre in Canada (IDRC)

An ecological intervention to interfere with transmission of schistosomiasis and other helminthic zoonoses became the basis for a 3-year IDRC project from 2011 to 2014 entitled 'Innovative Strategies for Sustainable Control of Asian Schistosomiasis and other Helminth Zoonoses through Socio-Ecosystem Based Interventions'. This multi-country and multi-institution project was shared among the NIPD, PR China; the RITM and the University of the Philippines, the Philippines; the National Malaria Center, Cambodia; Khon Kaen University, Thailand; the National Institute of Public Health (NIPH), Lao PDR; the Institute of Ecology and Biological Resources (IEBR), Vietnam; and the Research Institute for Aquaculture, Vietnam. Other collaborators included Swiss TPH, University of Copenhagen and WPRO. Dr. Robert Bergquist, (previously with TDR) was an independent advisor.

The results were expected to be used as basis for developing a classification system for target endemic areas based on environmental and socio-economic factors. The general objective was to develop innovative strategies for the sustainable control of target emerging infectious diseases (EIDs) through socio-ecosystem based interventions. The special objectives were to:

1. elucidate the environmental and socio-economic determinants of transmission patterns of the targeted EIDs;
2. develop a classification system for EID endemic areas based on environmental factors (the physical landscape, land use/land cover, vulnerability to climate change) and socio-economic factors (demography, migration patterns, trading patterns, health behaviour, water and sanitation, poverty and vulnerable populations, e.g., ethnic minorities);
3. define a set of tools for the integrated, sustainable and cost-effective control of Asian schistosomiasis and other important helminth zoonoses which can be readily combined in a modular fashion to meet local conditions; and
4. test the overall and relative effectiveness of individual components in the multi-disease prevention approach of schistosomiasis and other important helminth zoonoses in different environmental and epidemiological settings.

Each study site focused on two or more diseases and each disease was studied in two or more sites. From the baseline survey, a classification system of each study sites was determined. A stakeholder workshop was conducted to design the intervention programme including the monitoring and evaluation tool. The last year of the project was devoted to evaluation of the intervention that included an analysis of cost-effectiveness and sensitivity. Classification into eco-zones into epi-zones was done according to analysis of remotely sensed images and based on the disease-endemic situation.

The place, the dates and the target populations of the intervention packages were identified and the eco-zones showed the ecological differences, while the epi-zones showed the difference in disease spectrum and animal species infected. Within the epi-zones, hotspots were identified from where risk factors, scales and populations were identified with intervention strategies and intervention packages developed. The disease cover is shown in Table 2.

The project was divided into the following phases: baseline survey in 2011; classification based on results of the baseline survey and strategy setting in 2012; intervention in 2013 and evaluation of the effect of the intervention in 2014. The project ran for 3 years and included the following activities: protocol development, training courses (country-level), stakeholder meeting, training courses (field-level), baseline survey, data management and database production, data analysis, annual report (first), ecosystem classification system, designing intervention strategies, intervention, stakeholder meeting, intervention implementation, annual report (second), evaluation, annual report (third) and final report.

Table 2 Overview of countries and diseases covered by the IDRC multi-country project.

Country	Province/state	Type of ecosystem	Targeted emerging infectious diseases (EIDs)
Cambodia	Kratie	River valley (Mekong Basin)	Schistosomiasis, opisthorchiasis
PR China	Yunnan	Mountainous (upstream Mekong and Red rivers)	Schistosomiasis, cysticercosis, angiostrongyliasis
	Guangdong	River delta (Pearl River)	Clonorchiasis, angiostrongyliasis
Lao PDR	Champasak	River valley (Mekong Basin)	Opisthorchiasis, cysticercosis, schistosomiasis
Philippines	Northern Luzon	Hilly and mountainous areas with lakes and water courses	Schistosomiasis, cysticercosis
Thailand	Khon Kaen	Plain with lakes and water courses	Opisthorchiasis, fascioliasis
Vietnam	Nam Dinh, Ninh Binh	River delta (Red River)	Clonorchiasis, fascioliasis

Results of the project showed that the ecosystem perspective includes transdisciplinarity which integrates the perspectives of all relevant expertise; participation of the stakeholders in research project and understanding equity in the roles of different groups in the community. Lessons from the project include the recognition that the ecosystem of the region is taking responsibility for the helminth transmission and therefore there is a need for a classification system and identification of the hotspots. The helminths identified as problems in the region include cysticercosis/taeniasis, echinococcosis, FBTs (clonorchiasis, fascioliasis, opisthorchiasis and paragonimiasis), lymphatic filariasis, schistosomiasis and STHs. Three clustered zones were identified corresponding to specific helminth groupings. Recognition of social factors linked to local customs such as the food culture and unhealthy behaviour were found to contribute to the difficulty of helminthiasis control. The project confirmed that livestock takes a leading role in helminthiasis transmission (infection and re-infection). Higher re-infection was observed both in humans and livestock, and the lack of multi-sectoral cooperation was also noted.

Information Education Communication (IEC) effectiveness in the control of helminthiasis transmission was difficult to measure. There is no information on economic loss and disease burden, and there is no established model in the delivery of IEC materials leading to a serious situation on liver fluke infections and cholangiocarcinoma. Children, women and minority are vulnerable populations to helminth infections. Children are sensitive population of new infection while women should be targeted population of intervention. It is essential to keep a transdisciplinary team on surveillance and response to emerging infectious diseases (EIDs) in the region. There is however a lack of professional teams with transdisciplinary and EcoHealth knowledge. There is a weak capacity on quick response to EIDs.

Progress reports were given by the participating RNAS$^+$ member countries in the regular RNAS$^+$ meetings. RNAS$^+$ members also presented papers during the fourth Biennial Conference of International Association for Ecology and Health on October 15–18, 2012 in Kunming, China. Final results of the project were also presented in specific sessions of the 2014 EcoHealth Conference in Montreal, Canada August 12–15, 2014.

7.3 Control and elimination of helminth zoonoses in the Greater Mekong Subregion

A follow-up project was supported by the IDRC and dealt with the development of country-specific transformation frameworks to advance the elimination of schistosomiasis and effective control of schistosomiasis and liver fluke infections in the Greater Mekong sub-region. The project involved China, Cambodia, Lao PDR and Thailand.

The specific objectives were to:

1. understand the dynamic and interlinked drivers of schistosomiasis in Cambodia, China and Lao PDR and liver fluke infections in China, Lao PDR and Thailand;
2. design, implement, and evaluate a set of sustainable and cost optimized intervention strategies to support the control and elimination of schistosomiasis and liver fluke infections from the Greater Mekong sub region;
3. characterize the cost effectiveness of interventions targeting local drivers of transmission of schistosomiasis and liver fluke infections; and
4. identify and advance strategic opportunities to mobilize and generate greater investments for the control and elimination of helminth associated diseases across China and Southeast Asia.

The proposed activities designed to achieve these objectives are liver fluke countrywide mapping, annual MDAs, survey to determine infection status in humans, determination of the role of animal reservoir hosts in maintaining transmission, health education to promote control of targeted diseases and importance of water, sanitation and hygiene (WaSH), monthly meeting with villages team, review and analysis of the datasets of IDRC Phase I and cost effectiveness analysis of the intervention tools for targeted diseases in each study sites. Progress reports have been produced by the RNAS$^+$ member countries involved in this project.

8. Global engagements: International stakeholders

The overarching purpose of RNAS$^+$ is to strengthen collaboration among researchers, academe and control authorities in the regional endemic countries. From its humble beginning of a small forum designed for information exchange about research and experiences for the control of schistosomiasis in the Philippines and PR China, the network has gradually expanded its membership and scope to include not only zoonotic helminths but NTDs in general. Further expansion of this plan came as an offshoot of the workshop in 1998 when 70 scientists and representatives from the various control authorities gathered in Wuxi, PR China and planned the beginning of a network based on intersectoral, inter-regional and international collaboration for research, surveillance and control of schistosomiasis japonica.

From the very start, TDR provided the needed resources to gather experts from the Philippines, PRC, Indonesia and technical advisers from the United States, Australia, Denmark, and WHO among others. In its 20 years of existence, the following collaborators have continued to provide not only technical assistance or expertise but even material resources to keep the annual meetings of the network going.

- Australia: The Queensland Institute of Medical Research (QIMR)
- Switzerland: The Swiss TPH
- Denmark: The WHO/FAO Collaborating Center for Parasitic Zoonoses and DBL Center for Health Research and Development, University of Copenhagen
- Italy: Geospatial Health journal
- USA: Louisiana State University
- Control of Neglected Tropical Diseases, WHO
- WHO Regional Office for Western Pacific (WPRO)
- WHO Regional Office for Southeast Asia (SERO)
- UNICEF/UNDP/World Bank Special Programme for Research and Training in Tropical Diseases (TDR)
- The International Society of Geospatial Health (GnosisGIS)

Collaborations with the countries and institutions mentioned above strengthened as RNAS$^+$ continued to respond to the challenges involving various aspects of schistosomiasis initially and the network's other target diseases and then NTDs eventually. Aside from funding from TDR and WHO for early research projects of RNAS$^+$, IDRC injected research funds for a 3-year project in 2011–2014 involving several countries and several diseases for the purpose of developing innovative EcoHealth-based strategies for the control of the RNAS$^+$ target diseases in several member countries. IDRC sustained funding for another 3-year project involving countries along the lower Mekong Basin to continue developing control strategies for endemic diseases in these countries. RNAS$^+$ also established and maintained linkages with other networks such as RNSA in Africa, the Cysticercosis Working Group in eastern and southern Africa (CWGESA) and the *International* Society of *Geospatial Health* by developing and conducting joint training activities and attendance in each others' meetings.

The successful multi-country and multi-disease researches of RNAS$^+$ prove that RNAS$^+$ is now recognized for its ability to undertake such complex applied and operational researches needed to address the various challenges posed by schistosomiasis and other target diseases of RNAS$^+$. As scientists, researchers, academics work closer with control authorities elimination of these diseases is slowly getting nearer and within reach. Sustaining this linkage is a must to eventually reach the goal of elimination and beyond. RNAS$^+$ can boast of the following strengths for this objective:

1. strong collaboration in the regional research area that has successfully attracted a considerable number of experts on research and control
2. presence of experts in various areas who can improve and promote both research and control (For example, RNAS$^+$ includes more than 30 global experts who specialize on development of better diagnostics, vaccine and GIS-supported epidemiology.)
3. RNAS$^+$ has been successful in translating research output to field application (For example, RNAS$^+$ has undertaken development and evaluation of various control strategies for helminth infections while experts have the capacity to develop training packages on GIS applications, diagnostic tools, implementation and evaluation of health metrics and molecular biology research.)
4. setting up of a robust platform that is capable of advancing the mechanisms of sharing information through its website, databases, publications and meetings.
5. RNAS$^+$ has proved that it is capable of undertaking joint collaborative projects on operational research through multi-country, multi-disease using multi-disciplinary approach and involving different academic and research institutions in the region. Most importantly, experts who are members of RNAS$^+$ are also linked with control programmes of the endemic member countries in the region.

References

Cairo Working Group, 1992. The use of diagnostic ultra-sound in schistosomiasis—attempts at standardization ofmethodology. Acta Trop. 51, 15–28.

Cross, E.R., Perrine, R., Sheffield, C., 1984. Predicting areas endemic for schistosomiasis using weather variables and a Landsat database. Mil. Med. 149, 542–544.

Leonardo, L.R., Bergquist, R., 2002 Oct. Regional network on Asian schistosomiasis. Trends Parasitol. 18 (10), 434–436.

Li, Y.S., Kardorff, R., Richter, J., Sun, K.Y., Zhou, H., McManus, D.P., Hatz, C., 2004 Oct. Ultrasound organometry: the importance of body height adjusted normal ranges in assessing liver and spleen parameters among Chinese subjects with Schistosoma japonicum infection. Acta Trop. 92 (2), 133–138.

McGarvey, S.T., Zhou, X.N., Willingham III, A.L., Feng, Z., Olveda, R., 1999. The epidemiology and host-parasite relationships of *Schistosoma japonica* in definitive hosts. Parasitol. Today 15, 214–215.

Olveda, R., Leonardo, L., Zheng, F., Sripa, B., Bergquist, R., Zhou, X.N., 2010. Coordinating research on neglected parasitic diseases in Southeast Asia through networking. Adv. Parasitol. 72, 55–77. https://doi.org/10.1016/S0065-308X(10)72003-0.

Sripa, B., Tangkawattana, S., Sangnikul, T., 2017. The Lawa model: a sustainable, integrated opisthorchiasis control program using the EcoHealth approach in the Lawa Lake region of Thailand. Parasitol. Int. 66 (4), 346–354. https://doi.org/10.1016/j.parint.2016.11.013.
TDR, 1996. Ultrasound in schistosomiasis: a practical guide to the standardized use of ultrasonography for the assessment of schistosomiasis-related morbidity - Second International Workshop October 22—26, 1996, Niamey, Niger. Available at https://www.researchgate.net/publication/263088278_ULTRASOUND_IN_SCHISTOSOMIASIS_A_Practical_Guide_to_the_Standardized_Use_of_Ultrasonography_for_the_Assessment_of_Schistosomiasis-related_Morbidity_UNDPWorld_BankWHO_Special_Programme_for_Research_Trai [accessed Jun 14 2019].
Zhou, X., Acosta, L., Willingham 3rd, A.L., Leonardo, L.R., Minggang, C., Aligui, G., Zheng, F., Olveda, R., 2002. Regional network for research, surveillance and control of Asian schistosomiasis (RNAS). Acta Trop. 82 (2), 305–311.
Zhou, X.N., Ohta, N., Utzinger, J., Bergquist, R., Olveda, R.M., 2008. RNAS(+): a win-win collaboration to combat neglected tropical diseases in Southeast Asia. Parasitol. Int. 57 (3), 243–245. https://doi.org/10.1016/j.parint.2008.04.001.
Zhou, X.N., Wayling, S., Bergquist, R., 2010. Concepts in research capabilities strengthening positive experiences of network approaches by TDR in the People's Republic of China and eastern Asia. Adv. Parasitol. 73, 1–19. https://doi.org/10.1016/S0065-308X(10)73001-3.
Zhu, Y., He, W., Liang, Y., Xu, M., Yu, C., Hua, W., Chao, G., 2002. Development of a rapid, simple dipstick dye immunoassay for schistosomiasis diagnosis. J. Immunol. Methods 266 (1–2), 1–5.
Zhu, Y.C., Socheat, D., Bounlu, K., Liang, Y.S., Sinuon, M., Insisiengmay, S., He, W., Xu, M., Shi, W.Z., Bergquist, R., 2005. Application of dipstick dye immunoassay (DDIA) kit for the diagnosis of schistosomiasis mekongi. Acta Trop. 96 (2–3), 137–141.

CHAPTER TWO

Collaborative RNAS$^+$ research: Priorities and outcomes

Lydia Leonardo[a], Robert Bergquist[b,*], Shi-Zhu Li[c,d,e,f,g], Shan Lv[c,d,e,f,g], Virak Khieu[h], Somphou Sayasone[i], Jing Xu[c,d,e,f,g], Remigio Olveda[j], Juerg Utzinger[k], Xiao-Nong Zhou[c,d,e,f,g]

[a]Institute of Biology, College of Science, University of the Philippines Diliman and University of the East Ramon Magsaysay Graduate School, Quezon City, Philippines
[b]Geospatial Health, Ingerod, Brastad, Sweden
[c]National Institute of Parasitic Diseases, Chinese Center for Disease Control and Prevention, Shanghai, China
[d]Chinese Center for Tropical Diseases Research, Shanghai, China
[e]WHO Collaborating Centre for Tropical Diseases, Shanghai, China
[f]National Center for International Research on Tropical Diseases, Shanghai, China
[g]Key Laboratory of Parasite and Vector Biology, Ministry of Health, Shanghai, China
[h]National Helminth Control Program, National Center for Parasitology, Entomology and Malaria Control, Ministry of Health, Phnom Penh, Cambodia
[i]Lao Tropical and Public Health Institute, Vientianne, Lao People's Democratic Republic
[j]Asian Tropical Foundation, Filinvest Corporate City, Research Institute for Tropical Medicine Compound, Muntinlupa, Philippines
[k]Swiss Tropical and Public Health Institute, Basel, Switzerland
*Corresponding author: e-mail address: robert.bergquist@outlook.com

Contents

1. Introduction 24
2. Epidemiological studies 24
   2.1 The Philippines 24
   2.2 Cambodia and the Lao People's Democratic Republic (Lao PDR) 27
   2.3 PR China 28
3. Morbidity studies 29
4. Immunology and vaccine development 33
5. Diagnosis 35
6. Prevention and control 40
References 45
Further reading 51

Abstract

Over the past 20 years, RNAS$^+$ has been generating research results from highly collaborative projects meant to promote and advance understanding in various aspects of schistosomiasis. Epidemiological studies in endemic countries like the Philippines, the People's Republic of China (PR China), the Lao People's Democratic Republic (Lao PDR) and Cambodia clarified the role of reservoir hosts in transmission and the use of spatio-temporal methods such as remote sensing and geographical information systems (GIS) in surveillance of schistosomiasis. Morbidity studies proposed factors that might

Advances in Parasitology, Volume 105
ISSN 0065-308X
https://doi.org/10.1016/bs.apar.2019.07.007

influence development of fibrosis, anaemia and malnutrition in schistosomiasis. Immune responses in schistosomiasis continue to be an interesting focus in research to explain possible development of resistance with age. Results of evaluation of candidate vaccine molecules are also presented. New diagnostics are continually being developed in response to the call for more sensitive and field applicable techniques that will be used for surveillance in areas nearing elimination of the disease. Several studies presented here show the insufficiency of mass drug administration (MDA) with praziquantel in eliminating the disease. Emphasis is given to an integrated control approach that can be accomplished through intensive and extensive intersectoral collaboration.

1. Introduction

RNAS, originally conceived to strengthen collaboration among researchers, academe and control authorities in the region and countries endemic for schistosomiasis, was later renamed RNAS$^+$ as it expanded to cover a spectrum of other target neglected tropical diseases (NTDs). The network provided critical research input that led to a better understanding of their epidemiology through intense collaboration among the national research institutes in its member countries showing that the network has achieved the critical mass needed to build capacity not only for more research but also for developing control programmes designed to meet current challenges posed by global warming, burgeoning populations and rapid socio-economic changes. This chapter deals with schistosomiasis presenting advances resulting from collaborative researches involving RNAS and RNAS$^+$ over the past 20 years.

2. Epidemiological studies

2.1 The Philippines

A dynamic model of *S. japonicum* transmission, incorporating the effects of infection intensity, age and sex of villagers in the schistosomiasis-endemic province Leyte in the Philippines, was developed by Riley et al. (2005). The results show that the differences in infection burden between villagers are caused by differences in transmission and infection as well as the huge potential impact of mass treatment of all humans, particularly on those with high-intensity infections and the variable effects of a sudden snail population reduction. The intensity profiles were very different in children less than 7 years old compared with older children and adults. The research group used intensity profiles for helminths to describe the population infection status, monitor effectiveness of control programmes and provide accurate data to validate transmission models (Carabin et al., 2005a,b). It was, however, emphasized that the poor sensitivity of the Kato-Katz stool test and large heterogeneity in infection levels across villages complicate these predictions.

An extensive snail survey conducted by Madsen et al. (2008) in the same endemic province of Leyte, showed that density of the intermediate snail host in the Philippines, *Oncomelania hupensis quadrasi,* was remarkably uniform across habitats such as streams, springs, canals and swampy areas and without significant differences between rain-fed and irrigated villages, though the prevalence of infected snails showed more variability among habitats. Later, Saijuntha et al. (2014) pointed out that the phylogenetic tree and the haplotype network indicate that *O. hupensis* fragmented into *O. h. hupensis, O. h. formosana* and *O. h. chiui* and *O. h. quadrasi*, though the time when this ocurred was not discussed. Furthermore, genetic differences between some *S. japonicum* isolates in the Philippines were shown to be genetically differentiated from the Leyte and Luzon populations, while the genetic structure of *O. h. quadrasi* populations from Leyte, Oriental Mindoro and Cagayan are significantly separated genetically. This condition has also been observed between populations of *O. h. hupensis* in mainland China, where the snail populations' genetic structure relates to geographic areas and correlates with differing shell morphologies.

In a cross-sectional study of the prevalence of intensity of infection with *S. japonicum* in 50 irrigated and rain-fed villages in Samar Province, the Philippines, Tarafder et al. (2006) showed that people who work full time in a rice farm had a higher prevalence of infection compared to those who do not. Irrigated villages were found to be 1.4 times more likely to have schistosomiasis than rain-fed villages. Results further showed that the passive treatment approach failed to control schistosome infection in this region.

Water contact was studied in detail in a five-year project, where Payne et al. (2006) used three tools in determining the frequency of water contact in four schistosomiasis endemic villages in the Philippines: (i) bimonth interviews; (ii) self-administered diaries; and (iii) field observations. It was found that the agreement between the different ways of measurement was poor leading to the conclusion that the way measurements are carried out has an important impact on studies involving water contact. This project also greatly elucidated the role of mammalian reservoir hosts in the transmission of schistosomiasis. McGarvey et al. (2006) attribute the persistence of schistosomiasis in many endemic areas in the Philippines despite strong implementation of control programmes to the association with infected dogs and cats. This finding is backed up by Fernandez et al. (2007) who report that, unlike in the People's Republic of China (PR China), the prevalence of schistosomiasis in water buffalos in the Philippines is low. Rats and dogs on the other hand show higher prevalence of infections. This finding in addition to the significant village to village variation in prevalence could possibly suggest different transmission dynamics in the Philippine compared to PR China.

The results of the study of Riley et al. (2008) suggest that the process of acquiring mammalian *S. japonicum* infection is more important than the process of snails becoming infected and that this explains the difference in the prevalence of infection between villages. The group also showed that the contribution of water buffalos to human *S. japonicum* infection in the Philippines is less important compared to that in PR China.

Carabin et al. (2015), in their study of schistosomiasis in Samar, the Philippines found that dogs, cats and rats play a role in schistosomiasis transmission with dogs and rats showing consistent effects. Rats were recommended to be good sentinel animals in this environment. It was further suggested that future genetic and etiological research be conducted to understand the role of other animals in transmission. The One Health approach, involving experts in environmental sciences, veterinary and human medicine, could possibly contribute to the elimination of schistosomiasis in human communities.

Leonardo et al. (2012) showed lowering prevalence rates of schistosomiasis in the Philippines in a survey using stratified two-step systematic cluster sampling in a national baseline prevalence survey conducted in 2005–2008 based on one stool Kato-Katz as diagnostic tool. The group warned against lowering the guard of control authorities because of reduced rates but instead to prompt them to dig deeper to unveil the more detailed situation of the endemic areas through more intensive local surveys to identify 'hotspots' of the disease.

Leonardo et al. (2015) reported in detail the schistosomiasis situation in two recently discovered endemic provinces in the Philippines. It is hypothesized that the snail intermediate host has existed in these sites for some time but was only discovered now. Migration of people from endemic provinces into Gonzaga and Calatrava brought in the infection and with the presence of the snail, emergence of disease was just a matter of time. Hydrological connectivity through irrigation and river networks coursing through various geographic locations can easily transport snails into previously non-endemic areas. The last 10 years unusual weather patterns (as gathered from interviews of locals) bringing heavy rains and floods most likely carried snails from higher to lower elevations near human habitation.

The study of Magalhães et al. (2014) revealed significant spatial variation in *S. japonicum* infection risk, suggesting that spatially targeted interventions like mass drug administration (MDA) could result in efficiency gains for schistosomiasis control in the Philippines. Results of the analysis show that in the three regions of Luzon, Visayas and Mindanao, males and individuals aged 20 years had significantly higher prevalence of *S. japonicum* compared with females and children <5 years. *S. japonicum* infection was widespread in the Visayas whereas it was much more focal in Luzon and Mindanao. The research group suggested that when financially possible, additional schistosomiasis surveys should be prioritized for areas identified to be at high risk but which were underrepresented in the current dataset.

The burden of polyparasitism in endemic areas of schistosomiasis in the Philippines was underscored by Weerakoon et al. (2018) who observed an unusually high prevalence of intestinal protozoan infections together with schistosomiasis japonica in individuals in Northern Samar, the Philippines contributing to the significant public health and socio-economic burden affecting this population. Such results further justify the implementation of integrated control strategies for intestinal parasites.

2.2 Cambodia and the Lao People's Democratic Republic (Lao PDR)

Results of the survey of Matsumoto et al. (2002) first confirmed cases of canine schistosomiasis mekongi in Cambodia proving that dogs are important animal reservoirs of *S. mekongi* in Cambodia. No schistosome eggs were found in the stools of other animals such as cows, water buffalos, pigs, horses and field rats in the five villages surveyed in Kratie Province. The study proposed that dogs could have an important role in transmission because of their high susceptibility to *S. mekongi* infection and ability to release mature eggs once infected.

The study of Shimada et al. (2007) confirmed for the first time the high susceptibility of *Neotricula aperta* γ-strain of snails from endemic areas in Cambodia to *S. mekongi* originally isolated from Lao PDR. They described three strains of *N. aperta* (α, β, γ) finding the α- and γ-strains to be common in the Mekong River, while the β-strain only appeared in the Mun River, a tributary of the Mekong River in Ubon Province, north-eastern Thailand. The γ-strain was the first strain of *N. aperta* shown to be responsible for the transmission of schistosomes in Khong, Lao PDR. Infected β-strain snails have not been found in nature so far, while naturally infected γ-strain snails have been found in Sdau Village along the Xe Kong River, indeed the only area thus far from where *N. aperta* snails infected with *S. mekongi* have been collected outside the Mekong River basin. The discovery of high susceptibility of *N. aperta* γ-strain snails to *S. mekongi* from distant areas may be a crucial factor in the endemic transmission of schistosomiasis to humans.

2.3 PR China

Epidemiologic studies in PR China recognize the importance of knowledge and awareness and the overall socio-ecological context in understanding presence and persistence of schistosomiasis in endemic areas. In spite of the high overall awareness of the cause and preventive measures of schistosomiasis, knowledge gaps remain about the cause and transmission of the disease among students and farmers in the communities. Zhou et al. (2010) in their study in Eryuan County, PR China identified also other key risk factors, such as the absence of a sanitary stall house for livestock and presence of living and infected intermediate host snails in close proximity. They recommend the use of a spatially explicit Bayesian, multilevel approach to better understand the eco-social determinants that govern schistosomiasis transmission in limited geographical areas, while the study of Yang et al. (2013) in Jiangsu Province, PR China illustrated the usefulness of spatio-temporal analysis in assessing the risk for schistosomiasis. This approach could further be relied on with respect to surveillance and response that should increase as control progresses from morbidity control to transmission control.

The distribution of snail habitats is critical in monitoring and surveillance of schistosomiasis. Wu et al. (2002) showed that remote-sensing combined with ground-based ecological data collection can be used to produce classified images, not only capable of identifying snail habitats but also monitoring the impact of annual fluctuations of key environmental factors. Zhu et al. (2014) developed an ecological-niche model that adequately predicted the snail habitats in the mountainous regions by integration of a set of key data: the Normalized Difference Vegetation Index (NDVI), land surface temperature (LST), elevation, slope and distance from village to its nearest stream. The research group concluded that this model be used for the prediction of *O. h. hupensis* presence in mountainous areas, where snail surveys are difficult to carry out.

An important study showing the possible emergence of *S. mansoni* in PR China reassessed, using morphological and molecular delimitation procedures, the identity and presence of *Biomphalaria* species in a southern part of PR China near Hong Kong (Habib et al., 2018). Results suggest that although *B. straminea* is the only abundant species, this still poses a potential risk of *S. mansoni* transmission in PR China, particularly in view of the increased exchange with African countries where the parasite is endemic. More studies should be conducted to understand the biology of this snail and its competitive capacity with other local snail species and to describe its range of expansion. Finally, increased surveillance of all entry ports and checking for any exotic species are recommended in order to reduce the likelihood of future introductions of potentially invasive species.

3. Morbidity studies

Although morbidity has generally been strongly reduced thanks to MDA using praziquantel, some studies indicate that interference with the development of morbidity is more complex than so. For example, hepatomegaly and pipe-stem liver fibrosis may continue despite intermittent chemotherapy (Wiest et al., 1992). In a subsequent study, this research group (1993) suggest that the natural history of schistosomiasis japonica in a hyperendemic community in China, namely on Jishan Island in Jiangxi Province in PR China is characterized by the persistence of hepatomegaly and schistosome-induced periportal fibrosis in adults in spite of a reduction in the prevalence of infection. In addition, Olds et al. (1996) noted that morbidity from *S. japonicum* infection appears unrelated to the intensity of infection. It is also observed to be more severe than that caused by *S. mansoni* infection in terms of liver pathology and stunting of child growth and development. Both hepatic enlargement and fibrosis can be reversed and prevented with aggressive treatment. In the Philippines, rebound morbidity after reinfection necessitates short treatment intervals between screening and treatment to ensure significant impact on morbidity. For these reasons, RNAS and RNAS$^+$ researchers have continued to study the mechanisms involved in morbidity development, anaemia in particular.

The complex nature of anaemia and the need for combined approaches to treatment in tropical settings have been made clear in a series of studies by two research groups in Leyte, the Philippines. Kanzaria et al. (2005) showed that only high-intensity infections result in significant anaemia. Their findings indicate mechanisms other than extra-corporeal iron loss that could contribute to *S. japonicum*-associated anaemia, possibly anaemia due to inflammation. This should be considered for interventions involving iron repletion. Friedman et al. (2005), showing that cases with high-intensity *S. japonicum* infection were 3.5 times more likely to have faecal, occult blood, came to the same conclusion.

Leenstra et al. (2006a,b), on the other hand, came to the opposite conclusion. Their findings underscore anaemia as an important manifestation of chronic *S. japonicum* infection, even in low-intensity infection. This research group also assessed the impact of reinfection with *S. japonicum* after treatment with praziquantel on the mean haemoglobin level, iron-deficiency, non-iron-deficiency anaemia and inflammatory markers. It was found that the main mechanism of *S. japonicum*-associated anaemia, that is operating also in low-intensity infections, is a proinflammatory cytokine-mediated chain the eventually leads to anaemia.

Adding further information to this question, Ezeamama et al. (2008) showed that co-infection of hookworm and either *S. japonicum* or *Trichuris trichiura* is correlated with increased levels of anaemia than would be expected if the effects of these species had independent effects. Results imply that integrated anti-helminthic treatment programmes with simultaneous deworming for *S. japonicum* and some STH could result in greater than additive benefit for reducing anaemia in helminth-endemic regions. Taken together these studies point to anaemia as a general inflammatory response, rather than, due to extracorporeal iron loss in chronic schistosomiasis. Therefore, iron therapy may not always be the most efficacious way of ameliorating this problem.

Aside from anaemia, other subtle morbidities associated with chronic schistosomiasis are malnutrition and stunting. Results of the study of McGarvey et al. (1992) show that the growth retardation as an effect of high-intensity of schistosomiasis japonica in children is independent of the influence of other parasites, such as hookworm. McGarvey et al. (1996) also show, in a study in north-eastern Leyte that schistosomiasis caused decreased nutritional status in children, which is partly responsible for the malnutrition and reduction in growth for age described in prior cross-sectional studies. Although schistosomiasis is associated with malnutrition, the mechanisms involved are not known.

Another study in Leyte suggests that *S. japonicum*–associated nutritional morbidity could also be partly facilitated by systemic inflammation (Coutinho et al., 2007a,b). Malnutrition could therefore be the result of a combination of anorexia, metabolic changes, and body protein redistribution, leading to cachexia. This implies that nutritional supplementation alone may not be effective in lowering nutritional morbidity in areas endemic for *S. japonicum* and should be combined with schistosomiasis control strategies.

Coutinho et al. (2005) conclude that, in children, adolescents, and young adults infected with *S. japonicum*, hepatic fibrosis is associated with impaired nutritional status. Early recognition and treatment of this type of morbidity can be critical because of the strong evidence linking malnutrition with the detrimental effects with respect to morbidity, mortality, cognitive development, reproduction and capacity for physical activity. The group further shows that even low-grade hepatic fibrosis is associated with significantly worse nutritional status. These researchers hypothesize that it could lead to malnutrition and anaemia through a systemic increase in proinflammatory cytokine levels, specifically IL-1 and IL-6—and possibly TNF-α.

In a prospective cohort study in Leyte, Coutinho et al. (2007a,b) found results suggesting an independent role for the Th2-biased cytokine responses to *S. japonicum* antigens in the persistence of hepatic fibrosis. Further results indicate that Th2 cytokines may play a role in the higher prevalence of fibrosis in males. Males showed consistently stronger Th2 cytokine responses to both adult worm antigen preparation (SWAP) and *Schistosoma* soluble egg antigens (SEA) than did females.

Fabre et al. (2011) suggest that the Tissue Inhibitor of Metalloproteinase-1 (TIMP-1) is a promising biomarker for assessing risk of hepatic fibrosis in schistosomiasis and, potentially, other infectious and non-infectious causes of liver disease. With the use of a multiplex assay that quantifies predictors and effect modifiers of fibrosis (FibroPlex), these authors (2011) show that individuals with detectable tissue inhibitor of TIMP-1 had a 3.5-fold greater risk of fibrosis 1 year after praziquantel treatment. Since TIMP-1 inhibits most enzymes responsible for collagen degradation, the results indicate that schistosome-associated hepatic fibrosis could arise from excessive inhibition of collagen remodelling. Fabre et al. (2011) are presently evaluating the performance characteristic of serum measures of the TIMP-MMP axis in a bid to identify patients who may be at high risk of hepatic fibrosis.

A review done by Olveda et al. (2014a,c) shows that eggs cause bowel lesions ranging from colitis to polyp formation. In the liver, granuloma formation and subsequent fibrosis involve immune responses initially mediated by Th1 and later by Th2 lymphocytes. As a result of severe fibrosis, there may be portal hypertension-related complications causing significant illness or death. Liver biopsy and imaging techniques such as ultrasonography, computed tomography (CT) and magnetic resonance imaging (MRI) can assess hepatosplenic disease for proper management. These authors also highlight new serum markers for the evaluation of schistosome-induced hepatic fibrosis, namely hyaluronic acid, collagen type III, YKL-40 and laminin. The utility of matrix metalloproteinases and inhibitors, and cytokines needs to be further evaluated. Because of the strong correlation between the expression profile of miRNAs and the disease status/progression, circulating host miRNAs can possibly become very useful biomarkers.

Olveda et al. (2014b,c,d) claim that significant morbidity is seen in about 5% of diagnosed cases. This includes enlargement of the spleen resulting from portal hypertension caused by hepatic fibrosis. Portal hypertension can further result in massive bleeding due to ruptured oesophageal varices and pancytopenia due to hypersplenism. This research group also report a first case in the Philippines of portal vein thrombosis in a 12 year-old Filipino boy with advanced schistosomiasis. The patient was admitted because of rapidly enlarging spleen post-praziquantel treatment. After undergoing splenectomy, the patient was eventually discharged in good condition.

Further work by Olveda et al. (2017) assessed subclinical morbidity from schistosomiasis in 565 patients, using the enhanced liver fibrosis (ELF) test for the first time as a potential screening tool for disease. Results of the study showed the short-term impact of praziquantel treatment on both the prevalence and intensity of infection, but less on established morbidity. Certain measurements such as higher TIMP-1 and hyaluronic acid (HA) serum levels, and an ELF cut-off score of 8 were found to be associated with the grade of liver fibrosis. Such parameters can be used as basis of physicians in identifying individuals at greater risk of disease. The group concluded that a high level of schistosomiasis-induced morbidity is manifested by subjects with signs and symptoms suggestive of the disease in a moderately endemic area of the Philippines where active community-based chemotherapy has been implemented for over three decades.

According to Olveda et al. (2017), hepatic fibrosis, which is the root of hepatosplenic schistosomiasis, does not reverse quickly with chemotherapy. Identification and treatment of individuals with hepatosplenic schistosomiasis should be done as early as possible to prevent disease progression and possible death. Programme managers can use serum fibrosis markers, particularly high TIMP-1 and HA levels and ELF scores above 8 as basis to direct limited health care resources for schistosomiasis control. If cost can be lowered to facilitate its field application, the ELF test may assist clinicians in assessing patients with heavy intensities of infection (>400 epg) and/or those with physical signs of advanced disease (e.g. MCL >3) in determining their risk of severe liver fibrosis.

Hirose et al. (2007) show that *S. japonicum* and *S. mekongi* differ in their oviposition behaviour in their mammalian hosts which would help clarify the difference in morbidity caused by infection with these two closely related *Schistosoma* species. Their study reveals that in mice infected with *S. mekongi*, 56.6–69.4% of total eggs deposited were found in the distal small intestine 9–15 weeks after infection, while in mice infected with *S. japonicum*, 48.8–71.8% of eggs were located in the proximal small intestine during the same period. Additionally, a significantly higher number of eggs were seen in the liver in mice infected with *S. japonicum* than in those infected with *S. mekongi* which could possibly explain the more severe liver parenchymal changes in *S. japonicum* infection as detected by ultrasonography. This study also indicates that sexual maturity of *S. mekongi* lags that of *S. japonicum* which explains the higher number of mature eggs in *S. japonicum* infected mice compared with *S. mekongi*-infected mice.

4. Immunology and vaccine development

Noting the presence of *S. japonicum*-encoded, mammalian-like receptors for insulin, progesterone, cytokines, neuropeptides, Hu et al. (2004) propose that host hormones or endogenous parasite homologues could coordinate schistosome development and maturation. Schistosomes are also known to regulate anti-parasite immune responses through inhibitors, molecular mimicry and other evasion strategies. Transcriptome analyses, carried out by this research group (2004) based on numerous novel genes identified from a large dataset of expressed sequence tags (ESTs) generated from *S. japonicum* and *S. mansoni*, provide the basis for a thorough understanding of the molecular processes involved in schistosome nutrition and metabolism, host dependent development, immune evasion and invertebrate evolution. From this study additional potential vaccine candidates and drug targets have been proposed.

Webster et al. (1997) investigated the effects of host age and sex on human antibody isotype responses to *S. mansoni* and *S. japonicum* soluble worm antigen preparation (SWAP) and soluble egg antigen (SEA), using sera from subjects from Kenya and the Philippines. Their results show similar trends between the two populations despite differences in host, parasite and environmental differences between the two geographical locations.

A study of Acosta et al. (2002) in Leyte found that children of the 5–14 age group are the most vulnerable to rapid reinfection with females found to be more likely to be resistant. There is a reduction in the incidence in older age groups (15–19) and a lower intensity of infection starting around 15 years of age indicating development of immunity. In a later study by Acosta et al. (2004), also in Leyte, results suggest that resistance may be associated with mechanisms directed towards a Th1 response, while IgE in contrast to other studies appeared to be associated with susceptibility in older individuals. It was hypothesized that in this population a Th1 response predominates, where IFN-γ could strongly mediate protection, of particular interest being the significant Th1-type immune responses elicited by rPMY, a well-recognized vaccine candidate against schistosomiasis. This study strongly indicates the importance of IFN-γ in protection. However, there are also indications pointing to antibodies, particularly IgG4, IgE, and IgA responses to SWAP, a preparation containing numerous potentially protective epitopes mediated by Th2-regulated responses.

The higher prevalence and intensity of schistosomiasis in younger individuals is believed to be consistent with either slow development of resistance or the requirement of host developmental changes for the expression of resistance. The study of Kurtis et al. (2006), also working in Leyte, discusses this age-related pattern showing that serum levels of dehydroepiandrosterone sulfate (DHEA-S), a marker for adrenal development, are elevated and associated with reduced *S. japonicum* infection and reinfection, even after adjusting for age and cumulative exposure. These results indicate that an essential property of host pubertal development facilitates resistance to infection observed in older individuals. DHEA-S has potent immunomodulatory activities, including up-regulation of Th2-driven antibody isotypes and down-regulation of proinflammatory cytokines. Whether DHEA-S facilitates resistance in humans through a direct anti-parasite effect or through an innate or acquired immune mechanisms remains unknown.

A subsequent study of Coutinho et al. (2007a,b) suggests that the puberty-associated rise in DHEA-S down-regulates proinflammatory immune responses thereby reducing malnutrition and anaemia in a population with high burden of chronic helminth infections. These results improve the present understanding of the complex relations between chronic helminth infections, inflammation, and nutritional morbidity which could influence other paediatric chronic inflammatory conditions. Such newly discovered regulatory mechanisms of inflammation-related nutritional morbidity further stress the importance of treating prepubescent children for helminth infections.

With respect to susceptibility of bovine reservoir hosts, Yang et al. (2012a,b) confirm that 'yellow cattle' are more susceptible to *S. japonicum* than the water buffalo. The disease in this type of cattle also manifests as more serious pathological damage than in other livestock. Immunological analysis suggests that $CD4^+$ T cells might be an essential component of the immune response associated with the infection and a switch from Th1 to Th2 type polarized immunity was only clearly observed in these cows. Such results can potentially be the reason why schistosomes thrive better and cause more serious pathological impairment in 'yellow cattle' than in the water buffalo. The absence of a Th1/Th2 shift from in water buffalos could possibly explain the mechanism of self-cure in this animal.

Rapid reinfection that occurs after treatment, attended by extensive residual morbidity, necessitates alternative control strategies, including vaccine development. Shi et al. (2002) developed two experimental DNA vaccines capable of inducing partial protection in water buffaloes naturally exposed to *S. japonicum* infection in the field. In this study, Shi et al. (2002) proved that the vaccine candidate VRSj28 induced a 44% reduction with respect to worm recovery and a 77% reduction of the numbers of miracidia hatching from faeces, while another candidate, VRSj23, induced 33% and 68%, respectively. In this connection, Jiz et al. (2008) demonstrated that Th2-biased immune responses to paramyosin, a myofibrillar protein found only in invertebrates, are associated with resistance to reinfection with *S. japonicum* in humans. Further studies of this promising vaccine have been delayed due to challenges in the pilot-scale production of schistosome paramyosin. This molecule has been extensively investigated as a vaccine candidate for both *S. mansoni* and *S. japonicum*.

Jiz et al. (2008) developed a pilot scale expression and purification scheme for recombinant full-length *S. japonicum* paramyosin which is expected to propel studies in further evaluation of paramyosin. Wu et al. (2017) in a follow up study conducted three vaccine trials to assess the efficacy of recombinant full-length paramyosin (rSj97) in protecting water buffaloes from infection. Lower worm burdens were recorded for buffaloes immunized with the recombinant molecule indicating that rSj97 is a safe and promising molecule for use as vaccine against schistosomiasis japonica in water buffalos.

5. Diagnosis

Sensitive and accurate diagnostics has a vital role in reaching disease elimination goals for schistosomiasis japonica, which to this day remains a major public health and socioeconomic concern in Southeast Asia. Given the progress achieved with intense prevention and control measures, the ability to quantify infection intensity and the use of non-invasive diagnostics are the requirements needed for effective, improved surveillance. In the Philippines, the nation-wide prevalence may be relatively low, while it can reach as high as 65% in some endemic areas. Kato-Katz stool examination (Katz et al., 1972), which is the approach used for surveys to determine prevalence, has been shown to lack the level of sensitivity needed in areas characterized as low-intensity infections.

Bergquist et al. (2016) have reviewed the diagnostic situation for the whole field of schistosomiasis, while Zhang et al. (2016) discuss the development and application of parasitological, immunodiagnostic and molecular diagnostic technology for *S. japonicum* in the PR China, also briefly mentioning diagnostic imagery, such as ultrasound and radiology. Zhang et al. (2016) observe that the diagnostic procedures used in the past may not be as suitable today, especially not in areas where control has shifted the situation to elimination and surveillance. They conclude that the diagnostic approach should be customized according to the diagnostic needs in terms of sensitivity and specificity required in a specific control stage, previously discussed for diagnostic approaches in general by Bergquist et al. (2009). In PR China, the most widely used diagnostic techniques are still stool examination by the Kato-Katz method and the hatching technique (Qiu and Xue, 1990), while immunological assays, especially antibody detection, are used for screening with the parasitological tests used to confirm diagnosis following a positive screening test.

Diagnostic tests developed to detect schistosome infection range from basic microscopic test to highly advanced molecular detection methods. Requirements for an ideal diagnostic test or set of tests include ability of the test to make an accurate diagnosis preferably performed once, cost-effectiveness in terms of labour, easy sample processing, cheap equipment and reagents. With the next goal being interruption of transmission followed by elimination, the diagnostic tool must be both highly sensitive and highly specific since the endemic areas are changing into areas characterized by low transmission, low prevalence and low intensity of infection.

In the past decades, Zhu et al. (2002) developed a rapid, simple immunodiagnostic assay for schistosomiasis based on *S. japonicum* SEA conjugated with a blue colloidal dye (D-1) produced in PR China and used to detect antibodies in the sera of schistosomiasis patients. The antigen–antibody complex was captured by anti-human IgG absorbed onto a nitrocellulose membrane dipstick by means of immunochromatography. Results using this dipstick dye immunoassay (DDIA) showed high sensitivity and good specificity for the detection of schistosomiasis. The assay also produce rapid results, is simple and cheap and does not require advanced equipment. It proved to be more useful for screening target populations for selective chemotherapy than other immunoassays, mainly thanks the easy handling and rapid results. The reagents were also cheaper compared with the enzyme-linked immunosorbent assay (ELISA) but cross-reaction between *Schistosoma* and *Paragonimus* remains a problem of particular relevance to Southeast Asia.

Zhu et al. (2005) used the same technique to screen for *S. mekongi*. An estimated 140,000 people are at risk of schistosomiasis mekongi with 80,000 in Cambodia and 60,000 in Lao PDR (Urbani et al., 2002). The results of Zhu et al. (2005) demonstrate that *S. japonicum* and *S. mekongi* have sufficient mutual antigens to allow the use of *S. japonicum* SEA for *S. mekongi* serology. Its high sensitivity (97.1–98.6%), together with the complete specificity observed in relation to non-infected, healthy people, show that a DDIA based on SEA from *S. japonicum* can be used to screen for *S. mekongi* infections in endemic areas. However, cross-reactions with other trematode infections still need to be addressed.

In Cambodia, Kirinoki et al. (2011) assessed an indirect immunodiagnostic ELISA method using *S. mekongi* SEA. Sodium metaperiodate (SMP)-ELISA was used for the purpose of removing the glycosylated epitopes which are responsible for false positive reactions. The results of this method were compared with those using conventional ELISA. It was concluded that SMP-ELISA improved the specificity and sensitivity of schistosomiasis mekongi diagnosis, and it is expected that this method could become a powerful tool for diagnosing this disease.

van Dam et al. (2015) assessed the highly specific urine-based assays for the schistosome circulating cathodic antigen (CCA) and the circulating anodic antigen (CAA) by re-examining banked urine samples from Cambodia ($n=106$) and the Philippines ($n=43$) using the up-converted phosphor lateral flow (UCP-LF)-CAA assay and the point-of-care (POC)-CCA urine assay. Results of the evaluation showed that the sensitivity of a single urine POC-CCA was the same as that of a single Kato-Katz thick smear examination, while a combination of both CAA and CCA assays had a sensitivity close to that of triplicate Kato-Katz.

A follow-up investigation by Vonghachack et al. (2017) compared Kato-Katz stool examination, antibody detection by ELISA with the urine-based CCA and CAA assays in areas endemic for schistosomiasis mekongi. In addition, sera were also tested for CCA and CAA. The combination of applying the CAA assay in both serum and urine produced the highest prevalence of schistosomiasis mekongi (43.2%) among the 377 participants. As expected, stool microscopy only showed 6.4% prevalence of the disease. This approach has been further investigated in both Cambodia and Lao PDR showing excellent results (Khieu et al., 2019).

The accurate estimation of the intensity of infection in the mammalian host is critical to the understanding and modelling of the transmission dynamics of schistosomiasis (Riley et al., 2005). Carabin et al. (2005a,b) determined the sensitivity and specificity of a filtration and sedimentation technique (named the DBL technique after the Danish Bilharziasis Laboratory) in various domestic and wild animals in the Philippines not only proving the technique to be valid, but also demonstrating an excellent level of sensitivity. The DBL technique was further deemed to be good for monitoring infection in animal reservoirs using at least two stool samples collected on two consecutive days.

Wu et al. (2010) examined stools from water buffaloes in Macanip, Leyte for *S. japonicum* infection by the DBL technique, the Kato-Katz technique, miracidium hatching, and a highly validated real-time polymerase chain reaction (PCR). Their results demonstrate that microscopic-based techniques intensely underrate the prevalence of *S. japonicum* infection in water buffaloes. These results necessitate the re-evaluation of the role of bovines in transmission of *S. japonicum* to humans in the Philippines. The study showed that coprologic technique seriously underrates the prevalence of *S. japonicum* in water buffaloes. Since buffaloes produce 200-fold more faeces than humans (50–60 kg/day versus 250 g/day), even those with low infection intensities can significantly contaminate the environment. Since all the eggs excreted by the water buffalo contaminate the environment, transmission to humans cannot be easily prevented.

Gordon et al. (2015) examined faecal samples from six villages in Palapag, northern Samar using the Kato-Katz method and a validated real-time PCR (qPCR) assay. In their hands, the qPCR performed significantly better than Kato-Katz in detecting schistosomiasis infection and could therefore be used in the future for surveillance and monitoring of areas where extensive schistosomiasis control has brought down prevalence and intensity infections to very low levels making elimination eventually possible. Diagnostic surveillance using molecular tools like qPCR can improve the assessment of the effectiveness and impact of integrated schistosomiasis control strategies. Countries nearing elimination of schistosomiasis can benefit much from the use of improved diagnostic techniques such as real-time qPCR and also conventional PCR as well as the tests for circulating antigens in monitoring low-intensity infections. In PR China, where the disease is on its way to elimination, a rapid and sensitive method for monitoring the distribution of infected *O. h. hupensis* is urgently required.

Tong et al. (2015) successfully used a loop-mediated isothermal amplification (LAMP) assay targeting 28 SrDNA for the rapid and effective detection of *S. japonicum* DNA in infected and prepatent infected *O. h. hupensis* snails. This is the first report of monitoring infected snails from field sites of low endemicity areas by the LAMP assay using pooled snail samples which in turn proved to be a more efficient way to screen large numbers of samples compared with previously reported PCR and LAMP methods. The LAMP technique has since been standardized for use with collated samples comprising up to 50 snails for rapid monitoring and used as an innovative tool for surveillance and response strategies in risk areas (Qin et al., 2018).

Considering the difficulty in diagnosing schistosomiasis by egg detection and because of the superficially low parasite load after MDA in spite of the parasite transmission rates remaining high, Kato-Hayashi et al. (2015) conducted population-based studies to test the presence of cell-free schistosome DNA in endemic areas in Sorsogon province, the Philippines. Cell-free parasite DNA refers to the potential presence of fragments of parasite-derived DNA in the host's body fluids. Results show that cell-free schistosome DNA is a promising diagnostic marker to detect active schistosome infection even in cases in which the parasite ova are difficult to detect because of treatment with praziquantel such as what occurs during MDA campaigns.

While the current cost of molecular diagnostics is expectedly high, this assay can undoubtedly provide a useful tool for detecting low prevalent/intensity infections, for monitoring schistosomiasis control programmes, case detection in travellers returning from schistosome-endemic areas, and in animal and environmental surveillance of schistosomiasis. Weerakoon et al. (2017) tested a novel droplet digital polymerase chain reaction (ddPCR) assay targeting the mitochondrial gene nad1 to detect schistosomiasis japonica. The tool was proven capable of identifying both prepatent and patent infections using *S. japonicum* DNA isolated from serum, urine, salivary glands, and faeces in a murine model. Trial of the assay in a moderately endemic area in the Philippines confirmed that the ddPCR method can be a valuable new tool for the diagnosis and surveillance of schistosomiasis, particularly in low-prevalence and low-intensity areas that are already approaching elimination levels. The assay was proved to have potential for monitoring in areas where disease emergence or re-emergence is possible.

The diagnostic tools for schistosomiasis that detect eggs in stools, urine and biopsy materials from infected organs, serological techniques that detect antibodies and antigens of different stages of the parasites or schistosome DNA picked up by molecular techniques are only capable of determining presence of infection and/or intensity of infection. They are, however, incapable of measuring the severity of pathology in the target organ nor the resulting complications. Even the clinical diagnosis is difficult because of the non-specific signs of the disease. In addition, the widespread use of praziquantel is expected to result in many changes in the clinical manifestations of the disease.

The review of Olveda et al. (2014a,b,c,d) shows the development of several generations of imaging techniques in the last 30 years that have been used in assessment of schistosomiasis morbidity. Ultrasonography has several advantages: it is portable and can easily be brought to where the patient is, significantly lower in cost and does not use harmful ionizing radiation. In addition, real-time images are provided at the bedside, and its capacity has been improved by the Doppler sonogram which can add prognostic information in addition to routine grey-scale ultrasound. Sites that may not be visualized by ultrasound can be detected by CT and MRI. While MRI does not use ionizing radiation the cost is much higher. Techniques in the last 30 years that have been used in assessment of schistosomiasis morbidity.

Chigusa et al. (2006) used ultrasonography to detect the presence of thickening of the portal vein wall and formation of meandering collateral circulation of the splenic veins in four groups of people who underwent praziquantel treatment during the period 1995–2012. Ultrasound images show that thickening of the portal vein wall could potentially improve with frequent praziquantel treatments. However, praziquantel treatment had little effect on established splenomegaly with meandering collateral circulation.

6. Prevention and control

In spite of the major progress achieved over the past several decades in PR China, the Philippines, Indonesia as well as Lao PDR and Cambodia, schistosomiasis remains a public health problem in many places and is also emerging in some areas.

Zhou et al. (2010) have reviewed the epidemiological status and transmission patterns of schistosomiasis japonica in PR China where the disease is geared at elimination within a decade, particularly taking note of the historical context and the experiences and lessons with the national control effort. It is revealed that an integrated control approach, implemented through intersectoral collaboration is critical, not only for reaching the goal of reduction of prevalence and intensity of infections but also for maintaining these parameters at low levels. There is strong emphasis on the necessity for innovation and an adequately flexible control approach to design interventions according to the changing nature and challenge of schistosomiasis control until the final state of elimination has been accomplished.

Williams et al. (2002) developed the first mathematical model on the transmission dynamics of *S. japonicum* which predicts that in the lake/marshland areas of the Yangtze River basin twice-yearly MDA is slightly better than annual MDA in reducing human prevalence. However, although praziquantel treatment in humans produces an immediate and large effect on human prevalence, bovine treatment or vaccination (blocking transmission) produces a greater impact with regard to human incidence in the longer term. Encouragingly, the model has been able to predict results of a human chemotherapy programme in Anhui Province with a high level of accuracy.

In 2000, the Philippine Department of Health implemented MDA using praziquantel as a cornerstone in the schistosomiasis elimination programme. In an epidemiological study entitled 'Schistosomiasis Transmission and Ecology in the Philippines' (STEP), aimed at measuring the effect of irrigation on infection with schistosomiasis, an eligible population of 30,187 residents in 50 villages in western Samar, was offered MDA in 2004. Tallo et al. (2008) found that this resulted in a far lower participation than expected. Existing individual and community factors were found to be related to participation but much more applied behavioural and social science research must be conducted to explain this result. Additionally, the results of the study of Ezeamama et al. (2012) to determine whether treatment of intestinal parasitic infections improves cognitive function in school-aged children, suggest that sustained deworming and simultaneous control for schistosome infections could improve children's ability to take advantage of educational opportunities in helminth-endemic regions.

Human MDA utilizing the drug praziquantel has been the mainstay of control in the Philippines for >30 years. Still, the prevalence of the disease within different endemic zones ranges from 1% to 50%. In many endemic areas, especially in remote hard-to-reach villages, severe end-organ morbidity is still present. In addition, infected children often present with subtle morbidities such as growth retardation, malnutrition, anaemia and poor cognitive function. The significant contribution of large mammals (e.g. water buffaloes, cattle) to transmission complicates control efforts and the zoonotic nature of schistosomiasis indicates that MDA alone cannot eliminate the disease. To confirm this, Olveda et al. (1996) investigated the impact of annual case-finding and chemotherapy with praziquantel in the Philippines over an eight-year period. The results indicate that any sudden cessation of current control measures would lead to a rapid rebound in morbidity. It was also found that subjects chronically exposed to schistosomiasis japonica develop age-dependent acquired resistance to reinfection pointing to the possibility of vaccine development as an alternative approach for control of this parasitic infection.

Olveda et al. (2014a,b,c,d) conclude that the dismal results of the use of MDA for schistosomiasis control just point to the complex nature of the human–schistosome interaction. Innovative approaches that can be sustained economically should therefore be developed. Olveda et al. (2014a,b,c,d) implemented a combination of human mass treatment, targeted molluscicides, bovine (water buffaloes and cattle) treatment + vaccination in 22 highly endemic villages in the province of northern Samar. The vaccine (a SjCTPI-Hsp70 construct) provided a 51.2% reduction in worm burden, a 61.5% reduction in liver eggs, a 52.1% reduction in faecal eggs and hatching of faecal miracidia in a pre-clinical trial in PR China. The success of the bovine vaccine including other integrated measures may eventually lead to sustainable schistosomiasis control and elimination in the Philippines.

In a cross-sectional survey in northern Samar, Ross et al. (2015) found that in spite of an active schistosomiasis-control programme for >30 years that included a MDA campaign in the last 5 years, the mean prevalence of schistosomiasis among 10,435 evaluated subjects remained high at 27.1% (95% confidence interval [CI] 26.3–28.0%), and the geometric mean intensity of infection among 2832 evaluated subjects was 17.2 eggs oer gram (EPG) of faeces (95% CI 16.4–18.1). The research group concluded that MDA alone was not adequate, neither for controlling the prevalence of intensity of infection nor for sustaining a reduced morbidity of the disease. Hence sustainable control of the disease will require an integrated, intersectoral approach that goes beyond deworming. The authors felt that insufficient drug coverage, low cure rates, poor drug compliance and lack of baseline information already before the start of MDA made progress unattainable. In addition, adequate monitoring and evaluation must be carried out once the programme is commenced.

Leonardo et al. (2016) state that schistosomiasis elimination in the Philippines is a tall order, and that a plan is needed for elimination where all the aspects of the disease, including a budget to support proposed activities, are considered. All strategies that include WHO-recommended operational components such as water supply and sanitation, environmental management, snail control and health education in addition to chemotherapy should be implemented in an integrated and inter-sectoral manner.

In PR China, Xu et al. (2015) noted that while schistosomiasis and soil transmitted helminths (STHs) have decreased significantly as a result of integrated control strategies and socio-economic development, other helminthiases such as clonorchiasis and echinococcosis have increased due to changes in social and environmental factors. The group recommends further studies to generate potential scientific advancements that in turn can be transformed into novel or improved interventions to accelerate the control of all helminthiases, not only schistosomiasis. The application of chemical molluscicides remains one of the most effective measures for schistosomiasis control.

Yang et al. (2012a,b) investigated the cost-effectiveness of molluscicide application in order to find an optimal management approach to control the intermediate host snail under acceptable thresholds recommended by the national schistosomiasis control programme. The study concluded that all stages of the control/elimination programme should implement mollusciciding to maximize cost-effectiveness. The research group felt that the use of molluscicide treatment once a year at least would be needed before transition from morbidity control to transmission control. Further, environmental modification to counteract snail habitats could be done as an ultimate option during the transition stage from transmission control to transmission interruption. During the latter stage, re-emerging snail habitats must be eliminated immediately.

In a recent review of the status of schistosomiasis in PR China, Chen et al. (2018) noted that schistosomiasis control has always been conducted with strong political leadership and support at the highest level of government. The 60-year history of the control and elimination programme was initiated in the 1950s by Chairman Mao Zedong when the magnitude of the schistosomiasis problem was recognized. He led the control programme himself calling for the elimination of the disease in all the endemic 12 provinces along the Yangtze River. Sustained progress was achieved thanks to the long-term political commitment and improved further with the improving economy. The authors state that achievements of this kind can be replicated abroad provided there is long-term support from local governments and the incorporation of social and economic approaches. The current Belt and Road Initiative project, aimed at boosting local economies with global health development through local import and appreciation of Chinese technologies and products, is expected to provide the steps necessary to achieve the ultimate goal of worldwide elimination of the NTDs, including schistosomiasis.

Ohmae et al. (2004) reported on schistosomiasis mekongi from the time it was discovered in 1957 to its present status where control efforts have been intensified. Both political and economic conditions delayed the implementation of proper control for the disease until 1983 when implementation of MDA with praziquantel rapidly brought down the prevalence of the disease. Serological diagnosis has been used to detect new but low-prevalence foci, while ultrasonography is used to evaluate remaining morbidity. The research group stresses the difficulty in controlling the disease and the need for complementing MDA with other appropriate control activities.

Muth et al. (2010) discuss the results of control activities in two endemic provinces (Stung Treng and Kratie) in Cambodia. Before 1994, baseline prevalence of schistosomiasis mekongi ranged from 73% to 88% with cases of severe morbidity like hepatosplenomegaly, puberty retardation and mortality. Starting in 1994, universal treatment with praziquantel was implemented with coverage ranging from 62% to 86% for 8 years which dramatically brought down the prevalence so that no new cases were reported in 2004 and only three cases in 2005. Mebendazole was also used to control STH infections which resulted in the reduction of ascariasis prevalence from 74.5% to 10% and hookworm infection from 86% to 40%. The report emphasizes how important political commitment is in achieving control of parasitic diseases also under conditions of minimal resources.

Muth et al. (2010) later reviewed the status of schistosomiasis mekongi in Cambodia and Lao PDR. Control programmes based on MDA with praziquantel combined with health education brought down the prevalence of the disease significantly. In Lao PDR, interventions started in 1980 but were interrupted due to political upheavals which resulted in resurgence of the disease. At present, a small number of foci continue to register high prevalence. There are still new infections in both endemic populations and travellers to these endemic areas. The review stresses the need for comprehensive guidelines for the elimination of *S. mekongi* and execution of bilateral efforts between Cambodia and Lao PDR.

Hisakane et al. (2008) evaluated the control measures against *S. mekongi* in Cambodia using mathematical models with simulations to evaluate the effect of universal treatment and targeted mass treatment using praziquantel to reduce the prevalence. Results indicate that control of schistosomiasis mekongi in Cambodia is possible with high coverage rate of universal treatment and targeted mass treatment. A successful preventive chemotherapy administered in the entire population of two endemic regions in Cambodia dramatically reduced the prevalence of schistosomiasis mekongi from 77% in 1995 to 0.5% in 2003.

Croce et al. (2010) in their study of the cost-effectiveness of the schistosomiasis control programme in Cambodia (1995–2006) found that, while the control programme exhibited substantial economical advantages, the expense exceeded the budget given by the Cambodian Ministry of Health. It was hence proposed to solicit assistance from the international donor community to avoid reducing activities.

The paper by Khieu et al. (2019) referred to earlier is basically a diagnostic field investigation. However, some observations made refer to the current status and plans for the elimination of schistosomiasis mekongi from endemic areas in Cambodia and Lao PDR. It was shown that the elimination of schistosomiasis mekongi in Cambodia is feasible if based on highly sensitive diagnostics because of the highly focal nature of the endemic areas. In fact, *S. mekongi* has the smallest distribution of all the six different schistosome species that can infect humans.

In spite of the significant progress achieved through MDA and strong multisectoral collaboration, elimination remains distant with current efforts. For the situation to improve, a much stronger multi-sectoral collaboration, establishment of a common database and changing the perspective to a surveillance and response approach, which all will require increased budget allocations.

References

Acosta, L.P., Aligui, G.D., Tiu, W.T., McManus, D.P., Olveda, R.M., 2002. Immune correlate study on human Schistosoma japonicum in a well-defined population in Leyte, the Philippines: I. Assessment of 'resistance' versus 'susceptibility' to *S. japonicum* infection. Acta Trop. 84 (2), 127–136.

Acosta, L.P., McManus, D.P., Aligui, R.G., Olveda, D.M., Tiu, W.U., 2004. Antigen-specific antibody isotype patterns to Schistosoma japonicum recombinant and native antigens in a defined population in Leyte, the Philippines. Am. J. Trop. Med. Hyg. 70 (5), 549–555.

Bergquist, R., Johansen, M.V., Utzinger, J., 2009. Diagnostic dilemmas in helminthology: what tools to use and when? Trends Parasitol. 25 (4), 151–156. https://doi.org/10.1016/j.pt.2009.01.004.

Bergquist, R., Van Dam, G., Xu, J., 2016. Diagnostic tests for schistosomiasis. Chapter 21. In: Jamieson, B. (Ed.), *Schistosoma: Biology, Pathology and Control.* CRC books, Taylor and Francis, pp. 401–439.

Carabin, H., Balolong, E., Joseph, L., McGarvey, S.T., Johansen, M.V., Fernandez, T., Willingham, A.L., Olveda, R., 2005a. Estimating sensitivity and specificity of a faecal examination method for *Schistosoma japonicum* infection in cats, dogs, water buffaloes, pigs, and rats in Western Samar and Sorsogon Provinces, The Philippines Schistosomiasis Transmission and Ecology in the Philippines (STEP) Project. Int. J. Parasitol. 35, 1517–1524.

Carabin, H., Marshall, C.M., Joseph, L., Riley, S., Olveda, R., McGarvey, S.T., 2005b. Estimating the intensity of infection with *Schistosoma japonicum* in villagers of Leyte, the Philippines. Part I: a Bayesian cumulative logit model. The Schistosomiasis transmission and ecology project (STEP). Am. J. Trop. Med. Hyg. 72 (6), 745–753.

Carabin, H., Mcgarvey, S.T., Sahlu, I., Tarafder, M.R., Joseph, L., De Andrade, B.B., Balolong Jr., E., Olveda, R., June 2015. *Schistosoma japonicum* in Samar, the Philippines: infection in dogs and rats as a possible risk factor for human infection. Epidemiol. Infect. 143 (8), 1767–1776. https://doi.org/10.1017/S0950268814002581.

Chen, J., Jing, X., Bergquist, R., Li, S.-Z., Zhou, X.-N., 2018. "Farewell to the God of Plague": the importance of political commitment towards the elimination of schistosomiasis. Trop. Med. Infect. Dis. 3, 108. https://doi.org/10.3390/tropicalmed3040108.

Chigusa, Y., Ohmae, H., Otake, H., Keang, H., Sinuon, M., Saem, C., Socheat, D., Matsuda, H., 2006. Effects of repeated praziquantel treatment on schistosomiasis mekongi morbidity as detected by ultrasonography. Parasitol. Int. 55, 261–265.

Coutinho, H.M., McGarvey, S.T., Acosta, L.P., Manalo, D.L., Langdon, G.C., Leenstra, T., Kanzaria, H.K., Solomon, J., Wu, H., Olveda, R.M., Kurtis, J.D., Friedman, J.F., 2005. Nutritional status and serum cytokine profiles in children, adolescents, and young adults with *Schistosoma japonicum*-associated hepatic fibrosis, in Leyte, Philippines. J. Infect. Dis. 192, 528–536.

Coutinho, H.M., Leenstra, T., Acosta, L.P., Olveda, R.M., McGarvey, S.T., Friedman, J.F., Kurtis, J.D., 2007a. Higher serum concentrations of DHEAS predict improved nutritional status in helminth-infected children, adolescents, and young adults in leyte, the Philippines. J. Nutr. 137, 433–439.

Coutinho, H.M., Acosta, L.P., Wu, H.W., McGarvey, S.T., Su, L., Langdon, G.C., A, M., Jarilla, B., Olveda, R.M., Friedman, J.F., Kurtis, J.D., 2007b. Th2 Cytokines are associated with persistent hepatic fibrosis in human *Schistosoma japonicum* infection. J. Infect. Dis. 195, 288–295.

Croce, D., Porazzi, E., Foglia, E., Restelli, U., Sinuon, M., Socheat, D., Montresor, A., 2010. Cost-effectiveness of a successful schistosomiasis control programme in Cambodia (1995–2006). Acta Trop. 113 (3), 279–284.

Ezeamama, A.E., McGarvey, S.T., Acosta, L.P., Zierler, S., Manalo, D.L., Hai-Wei, W., Kurtis, J.D., Mor, V., Olveda, R.M., Friedman, J.F., 2008. The synergistic effect of concomitant schistosomiasis, hookworm, and *Trichuris* infections on children's anemia burden. PLOS 2 (6), e245.

Ezeamama, A.E., McGarvey, S.T., Hogan, J., Lapane, K.L., Bellinger, D.C., Acosta, L.P., Leenstra, T., Olveda, R.M., Kurtis, J.D., Friedman, J.F., 2012. Treatment for *Schistosoma japonicum*, reduction of intestinal parasite load, and cognitive test score improvements in school-aged children. PLoS Negl. Trop. Dis. 6 (5), e1634. https://doi.org/10.1371/journal.pntd.0001634.

Fabre, V., Wu, H., Pond Tor, S., Coutinho, H., Acosta, L., Jiz, M., Olveda, R., Cheng, L., White, E.S., Jarilla, B., McGarvey, S.T., Friedman, J.F., Kurtis, J.D., 2011. Tissue inhibitor of matrix-metalloprotease-1 predicts risk of hepatic fibrosis in human *Schistosoma japonicum* infection. Int. J. Infect. Dis. 203, 707–714.

Fernandez Jr., T.J., Tarafder, M.R., Balolong, E.J., Joseph, L., Willingham, A.L.I.I.I., Belisle, P., Webster, J.P., Olveda, R.M., McGarvey, S.T., Carabin, H.T., 2007. Prevalence of *Schistosoma japonicum* infection among animals in fifty villages of Samar province, the Philippines. Vector Borne Zoonotic Dis. 7 (2), 147–155.

Friedman, J.F., Kanzaria, H.K., Acosta, L.P., Langdon, G.C., Manalo, D.L., Haiwei, W., Olveda, R.M., McGarvey, S.T., Kurtis, J.D., 2005. Relationship between *Schistosoma japonicum* and nutritional status among children and young adults in Leyte, the Philippines. Am. J. Trop. Med. Hyg. 72 (5), 527–533.

Gordon, C.A., Acosta, L.P., Gobert, G.N., Olveda, R.M., Ross, A.G., Williams, G.M., Gray, D.J., Harn, D., Li, Y., McManus, D.P., 2015. Real-time PCR demonstrates high prevalence of *Schistosoma japonicum* in the Philippines: implications for surveillance and control. PLoS Negl. Trop. Dis. 9 (1), e0003483. https://doi.org/10.1371/journal.pntd.0003483.

Habib, M.R., Lv, S., Guo, Y.-H., Gu, W.-B., Standley, C.J., Caldeira, R.L., Zhou, X.-N., 2018. Morphological and molecular characterization of invasive *Biomphalaria straminea* in southern China. Infect. Dis. Poverty 7, 120. https://doi.org/10.1186/s40249-018-0505-5.

Hirose, Y., Matsumoto, J., Kirinoki, M., Shimada, M., Chigusa, Y., Nakamura, S., Sinuon, M., Socheat, D., Kitikoon, V., Matsuda, H., 2007. *Schistosoma mekongi* and *Schistosoma japonicum*: differences in the distribution of eggs in the viscera of mice. Parasitol. Int. 56, 239–241.

Hisakane, N., Kirinoki, M., Chigusa, Y., Sinuon, M., Socheat, D., Matsuda, H., Ishikawa, H., 2008. The evaluation of control measures against *Schistosoma mekongi* in Cambodia by a mathematical model. Parasitol. Int. 57, 379–385.

Hu, W., Brindley, P.J., McManus, D.P., Feng, Z., Han, Z.G., May 2004. Schistosome transcriptomes: new insights into the parasite and schistosomiasis. Trends Mol. Med. 10 (5), 217–225.

Jiz, M., Wu, H.-W., Meng, R., Pond-Tor, S., Reynolds, M., Friedman, J.F., Olveda, R., Acosta, L., Kurtis, J.D., July 2008. Pilot-scale production and characterization of paramyosin, a vaccine candidate for schistosomiasis Japonica. Infect. Immun. 3164–3169.

Kanzaria, H.K., Acosta, L.P., Langdon, G.C., Manalo, D.L., Olveda, R.M., McGarvey, S.T., Kurtis, J.D., Friedman, J.F., 2005. *Schistosoma japonicum* and occult blood loss in endemic villages in Leyte, the Philippines. Am. J. Trop. Med. Hyg. 72 (2), 115–118.

Kato-Hayashi, N., Lydia, R.L., Arevalo, N.L., Tagum, M.N.B., Apin, J., Agsolid, L.M., Chua, J.C., Villacorte, E.A., Kirinoki, M., Kikuchi, M., Ohmae, H., Haruki, K., Chigusa, Y., 2015. Detection of active schistosome infection by cell-free circulating DNA of *Schistosoma japonicum* in highly endemic areas in Sorsogon Province, the Philippines. Acta Trop. 141, 178–183.

Katz, N., Chaves, A., Pellegrino, J., 1972. A simple device for quantitative stool thick-smear technique in Schistosomiasis mansoni. Rev. Inst. Med. Trop. Sao Paulo 14 (6), 397–400.

Khieu, V., Sayasone, S., Muth, S., Kirinoki, M., Laymanivong, S., Ohmae, H., Huy, R., Chanthapaseuth, T., Yajima, A., Phetsouvanh, R., Bergquist, R., Odermatt, P., 2019. Elimination of schistosomiasis Mekongi from endemic areas in Cambodia and the Lao People's democratic republic: current status and plans. Trop. Med. Infect. Dis. 4 (1), 30. https://doi.org/10.3390/tropicalmed4010030.

Kirinoki, M., Chigusa, Y., Ohmae, H., Sinuon, M., Socheat, D., Matsumoto, J., Kitikoon, V., Matsuda, H., 2011. Efficacy of sodium metaperiodate (SMP)-ELISA for the serodiagnosis of schistosomiasis mekongi. Southeast Asian J. Trop. Med. Public Health 42 (1), 25–33.

Kurtis, J.D., Friedman, J.F., Leenstra, T., Langdon, G.C., Hai-Wei, W., Manalo, D.L., Li, S., Jiz, M., Jarilla, B., Pablo, A.O., McGarvey, S.T., Olveda, R.M., Acosta, L.P., 2006. Pubertal development predicts resistance to infection and reinfection with *Schistosoma japonicum*. CID 42, 1692–1698.

Leenstra, T., Coutinho, H.M., Acosta, L.P., Langdon, G.C., Li, S., Olveda, R.M., McGarvey, S.T., Kurtis, J.D., Friedman, J.F., 2006a. *Schistosoma japonicum* reinfection after praziquantel treatment causes anemia associated with inflammation. Infect. Immun. 74 (11), 6398–6407.

Leenstra, T., Acosta, L.P., Langdon, G.C., Manalo, D.L., Su, L., Olveda, R.M., McGarvey, S.T., Kurtis, J.D., Friedman, J.F., 2006b. Schistosomiasis japonica, anemia, and iron status in children, adolescents, and young adults in Leyte, Philippines. Am. J. Clin. Nutr. 83, 371–379.

Leonardo, L., Rivera, P., Saniel, O., Villacorte, E., Lebanan, M.A., Crisostomo, B., Hernandez, L., Baquilod, M., Erce, E., Martinez, R., Velayudhan, R., 2012. A national baseline prevalence survey of schistosomiasis in the Philippines using stratified two-step systematic cluster sampling design. J. Trop. Med. 2012. https://doi.org/10.1155/2012/936128. Article ID 936128, 8 pages.

Leonardo, L., Rivera, P., Saniel, O., Solon, J.A., Chigusa, Y., Villacorte, E., Chua, J.C., Moendeg, K., Manalo, D., Crisostomo, B., Sunico, L., Boldero, N., Payne, L., Hernandez, L., Velayudhan, R., 2015. New endemic foci of schistosomiasis infections in the Philippines. Acta Trop. 141, 354–360.

Leonardo, L., Chigusa, Y., Kikuchi, M., Kato-Hayashi, N., Kawazu, S., Angeles, J.M., Fontanilla, I.K., Tabios, I.K., Moendeg, K., Goto, Y., Fornillos, R.J., Tamayo, P.G., JC, C.J., 2016. Review: schistosomiasis in the Philippines: challenges and some successes in control. Southeast Asian J. Trop. Med. Public Health 47 (4), 651–666.

Madsen, H., Carabin, H., Balolong, D., Tallo, V.L., Olveda, R., Yuan, M., McGarvey, S.T., 2008. Prevalence of *Schistosoma japonicum* infection of *Oncomelania quadrasi* snail colonies in 50 irrigated and rain-fed villages of Samar Province, the Philippines. Acta Trop. 105 (3), 235–241.

Magalhães, R.J.S., Salamat, M.S., Leonardo, L., Grey, D.J., Carabin, H., Halton, K., McManus, D.P., Williams, G.M., Rivera, P., Saniel, O., Hernandez, L., Yakob, L., McGarvey, S., Clements, A., 2014. Geographical distribution of human Schistosoma japonicum infection in The Philippines: tools to support disease control and further elimination. Int. J. Parasitol. 44, 977–984.

Matsumoto, J., Muth, S., Socheat, D., Matsuda, H., 2002. The first reported cases of canine schistosomiasis mekongi in Cambodia. Southeast Asian J. Trop. Med. Public Health 33 (3), 458–461.

McGarvey, S.T., Aligui, G., Daniel, B.L., Peters, P., Olveda, R., Olds, G.R., 1992. Child growth and schistosomiasis japonica in northeastern Leyte, the Philippines: cross-sectional results. Am. J. Trop. Med. Hyg. 46 (5), 571–581.

Mcgarvey, S.T., Aligui, G.D.L., Graham, K.K., et al., 1996. Schistosomiasis japonica and childhood nutritional status in northeastern Leyte, the Philippines: a randomized trial of praziquantel versus placebo. Am. J. Trop. Med. Hyg. 54 (5), 498–502.

McGarvey, S.T., Carabin, H., Jr, E.B., Bélisle, P., Joseph, T.F.L., Tallo, V., Gonzales, R., Tarafder, M.R., Alday, P., Willingham, A.L., Olveda, R., 2006. Cross-sectional associations between intensity of animal and human infection with *Schistosoma japonicum* in Western Samar province, the Philippines. Bull. World Health Organ. 84 (6), 446–452.

Muth, S., Sayasone, S., Odermatt-Biays, S., Phompida, S., Duong, S., Odermatt, P., 2010. *Schistosoma mekongi* in Cambodia and Lao People's Democratic Republic. Adv. Parasitol. 72, 179–203. https://doi.org/10.1016/S0065-308X(10)72007-8.

Ohmae, H., Sinuon, M., Kirinoki, M., Matsumoto, J., Chigusa, Y., Socheat, D., Matsuda, H., 2004. Schistosomiasis mekongi: from discovery to control. Paramed. Int. 53, 135–142.

Olds, G.R., Olveda, R., Wu, G., Wiest, P., McGarvey, S., Aligui, G., Zhang, S., Ramirez, B., Daniel, B., Peters, P., Romulo, R., Fevidal, P., Tiu, W., Yuan, J., Domingo, E., Nov, B.B., 1996. Immunity and morbidity in schistosomiasis japonicum infection. Am. J. Trop. Med. Hyg. 55 (5 Suppl), 121–126.

Olveda, R.M., Daniel, B.L., Ramirez, B.D., Aligui, G.D., Acosta, L.P., Fevidal, P., Tiu, E., De Veyra, F., Peters, P.A., Romulo, R., Domingo, E., Wiest, P.M., Olds, G.R., 1996. Schistosomiasis japonica in the Philippines: the long term impact of population-based chemotherapy on infection, transmission and morbidity. J. Infect. Dis. 174 (1), 163–172.

Olveda, D.U., Olveda, R.M., McManus, D.P., Cai, P., Chau, T.N.P., Lam, A.K., Li, Y., Harn, D.A., Vinluan, M.L., Ross, A.G.P., 2014a. The chronic enteropathogenic disease schistosomiasis. Int. J. Infect. Dis. 28, 193–203.

Olveda, D.U., Olveda, R.M., Montes, C.J., Chy, D., Abellera, J.M., 3rd., Cuajunco, D., Lam, A.K., McManus, D.P., Li, Y., Ross, A.G., 2014b. Clinical management of advanced schistosomiasis: a case of portal vein thrombosis-induced splenomegaly requiring surgery. BMJ Case Rep. pii: bcr2014203897. https://doi.org/10.1136/bcr-2014-203897.

Olveda, D.U., Olveda, R.M., Lam, A.K., Chau, T.N.P., Li, Y., Angelo Don Gisparil, I.I., Ross, A.G.P., 2014c. Utility of diagnostic imaging in the diagnosis and management of schistosomiasis. Clin. Microbial. 3, 2. https://doi.org/10.4172/2327 5073.1000142.

Olveda, D.U., Li, Y., Olveda, R.M., Lam, A.K., McManus, D.P., Chau, T.N.P., Harn, D.A., Williams, G.M., Gray, D.J., Ross, A.G.P., 2014d. Bilharzia in the Philippines: past, present, and future. Int. J. Infect. Dis. 18, 52–56.

Olveda, D.U., Inobaya, M., Olveda, R.M., Vinluan, M.L., Ng, S.-K., Weerakoon, K., McManus, D.P., Ramm, G.A., Harn, D.A., Li, Y., Lam, A.K., Guevarra, J.R., Ross, A.G., 2017. Diagnosing schistosomiasis-induced liver morbidity: implications for global control. Int. J. Infect. Dis. 54, 138–144.

Payne, G., Carabin, H., Tallo, V., Alday, P., Gonzalez, R., Joseph, L., Olveda, R., June, S.T.M.G., 2006. Concurrent comparison of three water contact measurement tools in four endemic villages of the Philippines. The schistosomiasis transmission ecology in the Philippines project (STEP). Trop. Med. Int. Health 11 (6), 834–842. https://doi.org/10.1111/j.1365 3156.2006.01638.x.

Qiu and Xue, Qiu, L.Z., Xue, H.C., 1990. Experimental diagnosis. In: Mao, S.P. (Ed.), Schistosome Biology and Control of Schistosomiasis. Publishing House for People's Health, Beijing, pp. 448–527. in Chinese.

Qin, Z.Q., Xu, J., Feng, T., Lv, S., Qian, Y.-J., Zhang, L.-J., Li, Y.-L., Lv, C., Bergquist, R., Li, S.-Z., Zhou, X.-N., 2018. Field evaluation of a loop-mediated isothermal amplification (LAMP) platform for the detection of *Schistosoma japonicum* infection in *Oncomelania hupensis* snails. Trop. Med. Infect. Dis. 3 (4), 124. https://doi.org/10.3390/tropicalmed3040124.

Riley, S., Carabin, H., Marshall, C., Olveda, R., Lee Willingham, A., McGarvey, S.T., 2005. Estimating and modelling the dynamics of the intensity of infection with *Schistosoma japo*nicum in villagers of Leyte, the Philippines: part II: intensity-specific transmission of *S. japonicum*. The Schistosomiasis Transmission and Ecology Project. Am. J. Trop. Med. Hyg. 72 (6), 754–761.

Riley, S., Carabin, H., Belisle, P., Joseph, L., Tallo, V., Balolong, E., Lee Willingham III, A., Fernandez Jr., T.J., Gonzales, R.O.'.N., Olveda, R., McGarvey, S.T., January 2008. Multi-host transmission dynamics of *Schistosoma japonicum* in Samar Province, the Philippines. PLoS Med. 5 (1), e18, Volume 5| Issue 1.

Ross, A.G.P., Olveda, R.M., Chy, D., Olveda, D.U., Li, Y., Harn, D.A., Grey, D.J., McManus, D.P., Tallo, V., Chau, T.N.P., Williams, G.M., 2015. Can mass drug administration lead to the sustainable control of schistosomiasis? J. Infect. Dis. 211, 283–289.

Saijuntha, W., Jarilla, B., Leonardo, A.K., Sunico, L.S., Leonardo, L.R., Andrews, R.H., Sithithaworn, P., Petney, T.N., Kirinoki, M., Kato-Hayashi, N., Kikuchi, M., Chigusa, Y., Agatsuma, T., 2014. Genetic structure inferred from mitochondrial 12S ribosomal RNA sequence of *Oncomelania quadrasi*, the intermediate snail host of *Schistosoma japonicum* in the Philippines. Am. J. Trop. Med. Hyg. 90, 1140–1145. https://doi.org/10.4269/ajtmh.13-0260.

Shi, F., Zhang, Y., Lin, J., Zuoc, X., Shen, W., Cai, Y., Ye, P., Bickle, Q.D., Taylor, M.G., 2002. Field testing of *Schistosoma japonicum* DNA vaccines in cattle in China. Vaccine 20, 3629–3631.

Shimada, M., Kato-Hayashi, N., Chigusa, Y., Nakamura, S., Ohmae, H., Sinuon, M., Socheat, D., Kitikoon, V., Matsuda, H., 2007. High susceptibility of *Neotricula aperta* gamma-strain from Krakor and Sdau in Cambodia to *Schistosoma mekongi* from Khong Island in Laos. Paramed. Int. 56, 157–160.

Tallo, V.L., Carabin, H., Alday, P.P., Ernesto Jr., B., Olveda, R.M., McGarvey, S.T., 2008. Is mass treatment the appropriate schistosomiasis elimination strategy? Bull. World Health Organ. 86 (10), 765–771.

Tarafder, M.R., Jr, E.B., Carabin, H., Bélisle, P., Tallo, V., Joseph, L., Alday, P., O'Neil Gonzales, R., Riley, S., Olveda, R., McGarvey, S.T., 2006. A cross-sectional study of the prevalence of intensity of infection with *Schistosoma japonicum* in 50 irrigated and rain-fed villages in Samar Province, the Philippines. BMC Public Health 6, 61. https://doi.org/10.1186/1471-2458-6-61, BMC Public Health 6:61.

Tong, Q.-B., Chen, R., Yi, Z., Guo-JingYang, T.K., Furushima-Shimogawara, R., Di, L., KunYang, L.-Y.W., Shao-Hong, L., Ohta, N., Zhou, X.-N., 2015. A new surveillance and response tool: risk map of infected *Oncomelania hupensis* detected by loop-mediated isothermal amplification (LAMP) from pooled samples. Acta Trop. 141, 170–177.

Urbani, C., Sinoun, M., Socheat, D., Pholsena, K., Strandgaard, H., Odermatt, P., Hatz, C., 2002. Epidemiology and control of mekongi schistosomiasis. Acta Trop. 82 (2), 157–168.

van Dam, G.J., Odermatt, P., Acosta, L., Bergquist, R., de Dood, C.J., Kornelis, D., Muth, S., Utzinger, J., Corstjens, P.L., 2015. Evaluation of banked urine samples for the detection of circulating anodic and cathodic antigens in *Schistosoma mekongi* and *S. japonicum* infections: a proof-of-concept study. Acta Trop. 141 (Pt B), 198–203.

Vonghachack, Y., Sayasone, S., Khieu, V., Bergquist, R., van Dam, G.J., Hoekstra, P.T., Corstjens, P.L.A.M., Nickel, B., Marti, H., Utzinger, J., Muth, S., Odermatt, P., 2017. Comparison of novel and standard diagnostic tools for the detection of *Schistosoma mekongi* infection in Lao People's Democratic Republic and Cambodia. Infect. Dis. Poverty 6, 127. https://doi.org/10.1186/s40249-017-0335-x.

Webster, M., Librandaramirez, B.D.L., Aligui, G.D.L., et al., 1997. The influence of sex and age on antibody isotype responses to *Schistosoma mansoni* and Schistosoma japonicum in human populations in Kenya and the Philippines[J]. Parasitology 114 (4), 383–393.

Weerakoon, K.G., Gordon, C.A., Williams, G.M., Cai, P., Gobert, G.N., Olveda, R.M., Ross, A.G., Olveda, D.U., McManus, D.P., 2017. Droplet digital PCR diagnosis of human schistosomiasis: parasite cell-free DNA detection in diverse clinical samples. J Infect Dis 216, 1611–1622.

Weerakoon, K.G., Gordon, C.A., Williams, G.M., Cai, P., Gobert, G.N., Olveda, R.M., Ross, A.G., Olveda, D.U., McManus, D.P., 2018. Co-parasitism of intestinal protozoa and *Schistosoma japonicum* in a rural community in the Philippines. Infect. Dis. Poverty 7, 121.

Wiest, P.M., Wu, G., Zhang, S., Yuan, J., Peters, P.A., McGarvey, S.T., Tso, M., Olveda, R., Olds, G.R., 1992. Morbidity due to schistosomiasis japonica in the People's Republic of China. Trans. R. Soc. Trop. Med. Hyg. 86 (1), 47–50.

Williams, G.M., Sleigh, A.C., Li, Y., Feng, Z., Davis, G.M., Chen, H., Ross, A.G.P., Bergquist, R., McManus, D.P., 2002. Mathematical modelling of schistosomiasis japonica: comparison of control strategies in the People's Republic of China. Acta Trop. 82, 253–262.

Wu, W., Davis, G., Liu, H.Y., et al., 2002. Application of remote sensing for surveillance of snail habitats in Poyang Lake, China[J]. Chin. J. Parasitol. Parasit. Dis. 20 (4), 205–208.

Wu, H.-W., Qin, Y.-F., Chu, K., Meng, R., Liu, Y., McGarvey, S.T., Olveda, R., Acosta, L., Ji, M.-J., Fernandez, T., Friedman, J.F., Kurtis, J.D., 2010. High prevalence of *Schistosoma japonicum* infection in water buffaloes in the Philippines assessed by real-time polymerase chain reaction. Am. J. Trop. Med. Hyg. 82 (4), 646–652.

Wu, H.W., Fu, Z.-Q., Lu, K., Pond-tor, S., Meng, R., Hong, Y., Chu, K., Li, H., Jiz, M., Liu, J.-M., Hou, M., Park, S., Lin, J.-J., Kurtis, J.D., 2017. Vaccination with recombinant paramyosin in montanide ISA206 protects against *Schistosoma japonicum* infection in water buffalo. Vaccine 35, 3409–3415.

Xu, J., Xu, J.-F., Li, S.-Z., Zhang, L.-J., Wang, Q., Zhu, H.-H., Zhou, X.-N., 2015. Integrated control programmes for schistosomiasis and other helminth infections in P.R. China. Acta Trop. 141, 332–341.

Yang, G.-J., Sun, L.-P., Hong, Q.-B., Zhu, H.-R., Yang, K., Gao, Q., Zhou, X.-N., 2012a. Optimizing molluscicide treatment strategies in different control stages of schistosomiasis in the People's Republic of China. Parasit. Vectors 5, 260. https://doi.org/10.1186/1756-3305-5-260.

Yang, J., Fu, Z., Feng, X., Shi, Y., Yuan, C., Liu, J., Hong, Y., Li, H., Lu, K., Lin, J., 2012b. Comparison of worm development and host immune responses in natural hosts of *Schistosoma japonicum*, yellow cattle and water buffalo. BMC Vet. Res. 8, 25.

Yang, K., Sun, L.-P., Liang, Y.-S., Wu, F., Li, W., Zhang, J.-F., Huang, Y.-X., Hang, D.-R., Liang, S., Bergquist, R., Zhou, X.-N., 2013. *Schistosoma japonicum* risk in Jiangsu province, People's Republic of China: identification of a spatio-temporal risk pattern along the Yangtze River. Geospat. Health 8 (1), 133–142.

Zhang, J.F., Xu, J., Bergquist, R., Yu, L.L., Yan, X.L., Zhu, H.-Q., Wen, L.Y., 2016. Development and application of diagnostics in the national schistosomiasis control programme in The People's Republic of China. Adv. Parasitol. 92, 409–434. ISSN 0065-308X. https://doi.org/10.1016/bs.apar.2016.02.008.

Zhou, X.N., Bergquist, R., Leonardo, L., Yang, G.J., Yang, K., Sudomo, M., Olveda, R., 2010. schistosomiasis japonica control and research needs. Adv. Parasitol. 72, 145–148.

Zhu, Y., He, W., Liang, Y., Xu, M., Yu, C., Hua, W., Chao, G., 2002. Development of a rapid, simple dipstick dye immunoassay for schistosomiasis diagnosis. J. Immunol. Methods 266, 1–5.

Zhu, Y.C., Socheat, D., Bounlu, K., Liang, Y.S., Sinuon, M., Insisiengmay, S., He, W., Xu, M., Shi, W.Z., Bergquist, R., 2005. Application of dipstick dye immunoassay (DDIA) kit for the diagnosis of schistosomiasis mekongi. Acta Trop. 96 (2–3), 137–141.

Zhu, H.-R., Liu, L., Zhou, X.-N., Yang, G.-J., 2015. Ecological model to predict potential habitats of *Oncomelania hupensis*, the intermediate host of *Schistosoma japonicum* in the mountainous regions, China. PLoS Negl Trop Dis. 9 (8), e0004028. https://doi.org/10.1371/journal.pntd.0004028.

Further reading

Blake, R.A., Park, S., Baltazar, P., Ayaso, E.B., Monterde, D.B.S., Acosta, L.P., Olveda, R.M., Tallo, V., July, J.F.F., 2016. LBW and SGA impact longitudinal growth and nutritional status of filipino infants. PLoS One| 11, e0159461. https://doi.org/10.1371/journal.pone.0159461.

Dama, G.J.v., Odermatt, P., Acosta, L., Bergquist, R., Dood, C.J.d., Kornelis, D., Muth, S., Utzinger, J., Paul, L.A.M.C., 2015. Evaluation of banked urine samples for the detection of circulating anodic and cathodic antigens in *Schistosoma mekongi* and *S. japonicum* infections: a proof-of-concept study. Acta Trop. 141, 198–203.

Hu, W., Yan, Q., Shen, D., et al., 2003. Evolutionary and biomedical implications of a Schistosoma japonicum complementary DNA resource[J]. Nat. Genet. 35 (2), 139–147.

Langdon, G.C., Olveda, R.M., McGarvey, S.T., Kurtis, J.D., Friedman, J.F., 2006. Proinflammatory cytokines and C-reactive protein are associated with undernutrition in the context of *Schistosoma japonicum* infection. Am. J. Trop. Med. Hyg. 75 (4), 720–726.

Olveda, R.M., Gray, D.J., 2019. Schistosomiasis in the Philippines: innovative control approach is needed if elimination is the goal. Trop. Med. Infect. Dis. 42, pii: E66. https://doi.org/10.3390/tropicalmed4020066.

Sinuon, M., Tsuyuoka, R., Socheat, D., Odermatt, P., Ohmae, H., Matsuda, H., Montresor, A., Palmer, K., 2007. Control of *Schistosoma mekongi* in Cambodia: results of eight years of control activities in the two endemic provinces. Trans. R. Soc. Trop. Med. Hyg. 101, 34–39.

Wiest, P.M., Wu, G., Zhong, S., McGarvey, S.T., Tan, E., Yuan, J., Peters, P., Olveda, R.M., Olds, G.R., 1993. Schistosomiasis japonica on Jishan Island, Jiangxi Province, People's Republic of China: persistence of hepatic fibrosis after reduction of the prevalence of infection with age. Trans. R. Soc. Trop. Med. Hyg. 87 (3), 290–294.

Yang, K., Zhou, X.-N., Jia, T.-W., Yang, G.-J., Wu, X.-H., Shi, X.-W., Li, H.-J., Steinmann, P., Utzinger, J., Bergquist, R., 2015. Eco-social determinants of *Schistosoma japonicum* infection supported by multi-level modelling in Eryuan County, People's Republic of China. Acta Trop. 141 (Pt B), 391–398. https://doi.org/10.1016/j.actatropica.2014.04.013.

Zhu, Y.-C., Socheat, D., Bounlu, K., You-Sheng, L., Sinuon, M., Insisiengmay, S., He, W., Ming, X., Wei-Zhu, S., Bergquist, R., 2007. Application of dipstick dye immunoassay (DDIA) kit for the diagnosis of schistosomiasis mekongi. Acta Trop. (96), 137–141.

CHAPTER THREE

Needs and coordination mechanism for capacity building by the RNAS+

Xiao-Nong Zhou[a,b,c,d,e,*], Lydia Leonardo[f], Juerg Utzinger[g], Shan Lv[a,b,c,d,e], Jing Xu[a,b,c,d,e], Arve Lee Willingham[h], Yan Lu[a,b,c,d,e], Don McManus[i], Shi-Zhu Li[a,b,c,d,e], Marilu Venturina[j], Remigio Olveda[j], Robert Bergquist[k]

[a]National Institute of Parasitic Diseases, Chinese Center for Disease Control and Prevention, Shanghai, China
[b]Chinese Center for Tropical Diseases Research, Shanghai, China
[c]WHO Collaborating Centre for Tropical Diseases, Shanghai, China
[d]National Center for International Research on Tropical Diseases, Shanghai, China
[e]Key Laboratory of Parasite and Vector Biology, Ministry of Health, Shanghai, China
[f]Institute of Biology, College of Science, University of the Philippines Diliman and University of the East Ramon Magsaysay Graduate School, Quezon City, Philippines
[g]Swiss Tropical and Public Health Institute, Basel, Switzerland
[h]One Health Center for Zoonoses and Tropical Veterinary Medicine, Ross University School of Veterinary Medicine, Basseterre, Saint Kitts and Nevis
[i]QIMR Berghofer Medical Research Institute, Molecular Parasitology Laboratory, Brisbane, QLD, Australia
[j]Asian Tropical Foundation, Filinvest Corporate City, Research Institute for Tropical Medicine Compound, Muntinlupa, Philippines
[k]Geospatial Health, Ingerod, Brastad, Sweden
*Corresponding author: e-mail address: zhouxn1@chinacdc.cn

Contents

1. Introduction 54
2. Need for capacity building 55
3. Improving capacity 57
4. Capacity building: Selected case studies 58
   4.1 Case study 1: Field training on veterinary schistosomiasis control and elimination 59
   4.2 Case study 2: Completed Ph.D. programme to be an outstanding researcher 60
   4.3 Case study 3: Internship training at WHO HQ on the improvement of research capacity on zoonotic diseases 61
   4.4 Case study 4: Achievements of EQAs on NTDs from 2012 to 2015 62
5. Capacity building opportunities 63
   5.1 Swiss TPH, Basel, Switzerland 64
   5.2 QIMR Berghofer, Brisbane, Australia 64
   5.3 RITM, Muntinlupa, the Philippines 65
   5.4 NIPD, China CDC, China 65
6. Conclusion 66
References 67

Advances in Parasitology, Volume 105
ISSN 0065-308X
https://doi.org/10.1016/bs.apar.2019.07.008

Abstract

For the Regional Network on Asian Schistosomiasis and Other Helminth Zoonosis (RNAS$^+$), capacity building with emphasis on modern technology with correspondence to traditional techniques was found to be a priority. This article summarized the actual needs of capacity building among RNAS$^+$ member countries and the working mechanism of capacity building during the last 20 years. The needs with respect to the RNAS$^+$ target diseases are highly correlated with the research priorities, since most problems with regard to the performance of the national disease control programme in the member countries are connected with inadequate capacity in relation to implementation of innovative research, epidemiological investigations, laboratory performance; and sociological investigations. The capacity building arranged through RNAS$^+$ platform includes short training courses, individual training in member institutions, e.g., supervision of Ph.D./Masters students; postdoctoral training; and internship training in institutions of southeast Asia as well as in famous institutions of Europe and the United States. In the future, capacity building will focus on platform design and technical standardization aiming at fostering research capacity in the future. Moreover, new training projects, such as massive online courses (MOOC) will be explored under RNAS$^+$ platform.

1. Introduction

With the development of Regional Network on Asian Schistosomiasis and Other Helminth Zoonosis (RNAS$^+$, *rnas.ipd.org.cn*), it was found the capacity building is of particular importance as there is a need to improve professionals from member countries in terms of technical performs of modern technology and also traditional techniques (Zhou et al., 2015). Particularly when the endemicity of neglected tropical diseases (NTDs) is reduced thanks to the well implementation of control programmes, it is an urgent for better diagnostic tools with higher sensitivity compared the traditional approaches (Osorio et al., 2018; Wang et al., 2018; Yang et al., 2019). For example, at surveillance sites, the level of endemicity might be underestimated due to lower sensitivity of traditional surveillance tools, such as Kato-Katz method. At the same time, the sensitivity of diagnostic tools varies due to different skills of the different professionals involved (de Sousa et al., 2019). Recently, more attention has been paid to performance quality, which has a direct impact on data quality and in the longer perspective the control strategy chosen (Ceccato et al., 2018). For example, the results from the external quality assessments of national public health laboratories in detecting NTD parasitic infections in six countries of the WHO Western Pacific Region, the overall coincidence rates for serum samples with titres of 1:40 was better than those for serum samples with titres of 1:20 or of 1:10.

Detecting low levels of serum antibody in schistosomiasis patients was problematic for indirect hemagglutination test (IHA) as it indicated low coincidence rates for serum samples with titres of 1:20 or 1:10 (<50%) (Lu et al., 2017). Therefore, external quality assessment (EQA) are needed to identify deficiencies in local laboratories in the endemic countries. Thus, there is a strong need to overcome and improve laboratory performance with regard to helminth diagnosis.

By understanding the abovementioned the needs for capacity building which directly relate to the quality of control programmes, the training activities arranged through RNAS$^+$ platform have been arranged every year. This kind of training activities are commonly linked with the annual RNAS$^+$ workshops, which are normally attended by professionals from each of RNAS$^+$ member countries (Zhou et al., 2015). This article summarized the actual needs of capacity building among RNAS$^+$ member countries and the working mechanism over the last 20 years.

2. Need for capacity building

RNAS$^+$ has provided critical input with regard to several parasitic diseases of Southeast Asia, in particular with regard to schistosomiasis research and other helminthiasis (Zhou et al., 2015). However, since various other helminthic infections are still highly epidemic in many areas of the region, and polyparasitism involving various helminthiases is common, it has been decided to extend the spectrum of the RNAS$^+$ targeted diseases into five focal areas, i.e., schistosomiasis, cysticercosis, clonorchiasis, opisthorchiasis and fascioliasis. Based on RNAS-organized workshop discussions there is a need for the development of new techniques, implementation of ecological, epidemiology studies, building of local technical standards and criteria, and the creation of new products and equipments (Olveda et al., 2010).

Capacity building for the RNAS$^+$ targeted diseases are highly correlated with the research priorities, since most of problems occur in performance of the national disease control programme in the member countries are low capacity in relation to implementation of: (i) new research; (ii) epidemiological investigations; (iii) laboratory performance; and (iv) sociological investigations.

By analysis of the research priorities, we found them closely correlated with the needs of capacity building of member countries. First, in the field of information management, the data handling is the basic requirement for the capacity building, which includes the research priorities on (i) documentation and development of health metrics useful in practice; (ii) promotion of geographical information systems (GIS) and remote-sensing techniques for the study of climate change and other applications. Second, in the field of laboratory capacity building that covers (i) encouragement of study of genetics and the immune responses against parasites to better understand the pathology caused and ultimately to apply for the development of a schistosomiasis vaccine, (ii) improvement and standardization of the diagnostic capabilities including development of new products, equipments and techniques; Third, in the field of epidemiological and sociological research, it needs capacity on (i) support of research on the impact of social determinants and economic issues on the epidemiology of Asian helminth zoonotic infections; and (ii) implementation research related to control strategies. Therefore, training activities in the abovementioned three fields were determined as training priority areas, including data handling, laboratory capacity, and epidemiological and sociological capacity in the field (Table 1).

Table 1 The relationship between research priorities and priorities of capacity building.

Research priority	Training priority
Documentation and development of health metrics	Training on surveillance data handling with regard to health information systems for infectious diseases
Impact of social determinants and economic issues on the epidemiology of Asian helminth zoonotic infections	Training on social determinants on burden of diseases, on cost-effectiveness evaluation and quick assessment methods for zoonotic infections
Promotion of GIS and remote-sensing techniques for the study of the impact of climate change and other applications	Training on geospatial techniques and spatial epidemiology
Encouragement of the study of genetics and the immune responses against parasites to better understand the pathology caused	Training on the genetics of parasite species, on diagnostic techniques, on vaccine development, and on molecular biology
Improvement and standardization of the diagnostic capabilities including development of new products, equipment and techniques	Training on standardization of diagnostic capacities, on new tools of diagnostics and control approaches
Implementation research related to control strategies	Training on implementation research, on ethical evaluation of research projects, on control strategy development, and on evaluation

3. Improving capacity

Capacity building arranged through RNAS$^+$ includes short training courses, individual training in member institutions, e.g., postdoctoral training and instruction how to obtain Ph.D. and Master degrees, as well as internship training in the World Health Organization (WHO), the Swiss Tropical and Public Health Institute (Swiss TPH) in Switzerland, the Berghofer Queensland Institute of Medical Research (QIMR) in Australia, the Research Institute of Tropical Medicine (RITM) in the Philippines, the University of Philippines (UP), the National Institute of Parasitic Diseases (NIPD) of Chinese Center for Disease Control and Prevention (China CDC) in China, and the Veterinary University of Khon Kaen in Thailand, Louisiana State University in the United States, to mention some of RNAS$^+$'s closest collaboration partners.

First, a total of 15 short training courses linked with the RNAS$^+$'s annual workshops show the major way to improve the capacity of professionals for the member countries. The contents of each training course are based on the needs and priorities with regard to capacity building in the member countries, which is decided by the RNAS$^+$ Board. Short training courses focused on information management and data handling, diagnosis with laboratory technologies as well as sociological research in general have been arranged, e.g., development of health metrics, GIS and remote-sensing techniques, molecular biology, immunological diagnostic tools, schistosomiasis vaccine development, standardization of ultrasonography, epidemiological surveillance, sociological research, social determinants and economic evaluation, improving control strategies, and also on ethical issues when doing research involving humans.

Second, >20 young scientists have been trained in institutions from member countries through the RNAS$^+$ platform, with training periods varying between 1 month and 1 year. For example, three young scientists from the Medical Research Department, Ministry of Health (MoH) of Myanmar were trained in the NIPD, China in the field of drug development and biology of vector, and two young scientists from the NIPD were trained in molecular biology at QIMR Berghofer, Australia. Further, >10 young scientists from China, Cambodia and Lao PDR were trained for the Ph.D. level in epidemiology, data modelling, drug efficacy evaluation, and NTD control strategies in Swiss TPH, Switzerland, and five students from China, Lao PDR and Indonesia were trained, either at the Ph.D. or the Master level received instruction at the UP.

Third, more than five 10-day training courses on scientific paper writing were held in RITM, the Philippines and NIPD, China in addition to the 1- or 2-day short training courses linked to the RNAS^{+} annual workshops. The 10-day training courses targeted to help young scientists to publish their scientific papers within 1 year posttraining assisted by course mentors were a major success. In all, >100 young scientists from RNAS^{+} member countries were trained in various ways.

Fourth, both the WHO Western Pacific Regional Office (WPRO) and the WHO South-East Asia Region Office (SERO) have provided internship opportunities for young scientist from RNAS^{+} member countries, and >10 young scientists were trained through internship programmes at these WHO offices at country and regional levels, and also at WHO headquarters in Switzerland. These trainees not only widened their views of global health but also improved their networking capacity and learnt coordinating skills.

Fifth, an EQA with reference to public health laboratories on the NTDs at the national level in selected countries at WPRO was organized by the NIPD, China in the period from 2012 to 2015. Two representatives of each participating laboratory were invited to NIPD to detect parasitic infections using the same prepared samples for serological tests (IHA and ELISA) and morphological tests (helminth egg detection by direct smear and Kato-Katz methods). Training activities were also given to those participates right after the EQA aiming to improve the NTD detection capacity in the region.

Abovementioned five channels of training have significantly improved the capacity of young scientists, both regarding research and control activities. This has not only provided an opportunity for the young scientists from Asia but also has made a remarkable impact on research and control for the development of RNAS^{+}. Also other means of scientific exchange were tried, e.g., study tours to China on schistosomiasis control programme participated by offiials from Indonesia and the Philippines to China. This not only helped the scientist to learn new techniques but also allowed Government officials to understand the importance of multisectoral cooperation in the control of schistosomiasis.

4. Capacity building: Selected case studies

Here are some of examples on capacity building to demonstrate that training really improves and develops young scientists for more far-reaching activities. This was done by, (i) a training course in China with focus on the field training on standardization of the diagnosis in schistosomiasis elimination stage; (ii) completion of a Ph.D. followed by postdoctoral studies at the Swiss TPH, in Switzerland in 2009. This scientist continues his research career at the Lao Tropical and Public Health Institute, MoH, Lao PDR on investigation of *Schistosoma mekongi* and other NTDs including foodborne zoonoses (FBTs); (iii) another scientist accepted an internship at WHO HQ on the control of zoonotic diseases control, which help him to finish his studies for the Ph.D. in China, and (iv) EQAs achievements with respect to the NTDs in multi-countries.

4.1 Case study 1: Field training on veterinary schistosomiasis control and elimination

Schistosomiasis japonica is zoonotic disease, endemic in three countries in oriental Asia, i.e., China, Philippines and Indonesia. Except human beings, >40 mammalian species serve as reservoir host of *S. japonica*. China has been progressing well by using comprehensive strategies in the control and elimination of the disease, including control and elimination of human and animal schistosomiasis. In the Philippines and Indonesia, control and elimination of human schistosomiasis has been implemented since early last century. Progress in the control of endemicity was made and resulted in a lowered incidence of cases and high-intensity infections, as well as improved programmes aiming to eliminate schistosomiasis. However, animal schistosomiasis represents a challenge that most be curtailed. It is felt useful to promote the activities to transferring of China's experience and technologies on domestic animal schistosomiasis control to Southeast Asian countries. To that end, NIPD held a training course on domestic animal schistosomiasis control and elimination from March 27 to March 31, 2017. >40 trainees from the Philippine Animal Husbandry Bureau, the Indonesian Agricultural University and also Anhui Province, China participated. The training course was conducted based on theoretical knowledge and practical experiences on animal schistosomiasis, including training on (i) review of strategies and approaches of schistosomiasis control programme in PR China, (ii) diagnosis of animal schistosomiasis, (iii) treatment on animal schistosomiasis, (iv) field practice on sample collection and animal schistosomiasis survey, (v) demonstration and laboratory practice on immunodiagnosis and parasitological examination.

The training course lasted 5 days with the components of theoretical teaching, on-site investigation and laboratory practice. The first part of the training course was held at NIPD in Shanghai to introduce the experience of the Chinese national schistosomiasis control and elimination programme, with emphasis on the evolution of strategies and technical guidelines of schistosomiasis control and elimination, schistosomiasis surveillance system and reference laboratory network. The second part of the course took place in the field in the schistosomiasis control station of Ruichang City, Jiangxi Province. Eight experts from various Chinese institute of veterinary medicine gave theoretical lectures, including introduction of Chinese experience in animal schistosomiasis control and surveillance of domestic animal schistosomiasis, immunological diagnostic techniques and treatment of schistosomiasis in livestock, etc. Then the trainees conducted on-site practice and laboratory detection of schistosomiasis in livestock, including collecting bovine stool and blood samples, performing IHA, colloidal gold test and hatching method for detection of the schistosome miracidium. All trainees visited the endemic fields, including snail infested areas, conducting health education on schistosomiasis in the community of Ruichang. The training course enabled students to truly apply what they had learned in the endemic areas of schistosomiasis. Through the training, the exchange of knowledge on animal schistosomiasis between scientists from China and Southeast Asia as well as the transformation of the Chinese experience in technologies in schistosomiasis control and elimination were promoted.

4.2 Case study 2: Completed Ph.D. programme to be an outstanding researcher

A Lao medical doctor and epidemiologist first attended the RNAS$^+$ annual workshop held in Lao PDR in 2003 during his Master programme in Tropical Medicine and International Health. After his participation, he realized that the RNAS$^+$ can bring researchers, health professionals and policy makers together for discussing, sharing, exchanging ideas and updating information regarding the research, control and surveillance on priority NTDs in the region, e.g., Asian schistosomiasis and other food-borne zoonoses, which might enhance control activities in the member countries. In 2005, he started his Ph.D. studies at the Swiss TPH and continued also joining RNAS$^+$ training courses, e.g., GIS training in Lijiang, China in 2006 and the manuscript writing workshop in Manila, the Philippines in 2007. He returned to Lao PDR in 2009 after his Ph.D. and engaged in the research work at the Lao Tropical and Public health Institute, MoH, Vientiane Capital, Lao PDR. He became an outstanding researcher in the field of tropical health, working diseases such as schistosomiasis, opisthorchiasis, soil-transmitted helminthiases (STHs) focusing on epidemiology, parasitology, diagnosis, morbidity and treatment. Importantly, he was also involved in the early stages of the successful research project entitled "Eco-health emerging diseases in Southeast Asia (EcoEIDs)" led by $RNAS^+$ and supported by International Development Research Center (IDRC), Canada. In this project, he was one of the leading researchers moving project implementation into the successful outcomes, which resulted in IDRC extending this reach project with another 3 years.

A alongside the success with $RNAS^+$ integration, he was also recognized as an outstanding researcher in his field by Geigy Foundation, Switzerland and has received the Geigy Award in 2014, which is the first Asian scientist to receive this award.

4.3 Case study 3: Internship training at WHO HQ on the improvement of research capacity on zoonotic diseases

One Chinese researcher working in the Department of Soil and Food-borne Parasitic Diseases, NIPD received a 6 months' internship in the Department of Neglected Tropic Diseases, WHO in Geneva, Switzerland between August 2017 and January 2018. Owing to the participation in four kinds of work, his capacity in control of the NTDs improved significantly.

He first participated in the establishment of Diagnosis and Treatment Guidelines for *Taenia solium* with special reference to neurocysticercosis (NCC). He helped extracting information and write the recommendations from the systematic reviews provided by international experts. Through this work, he learned the process how to establish a set of guidelines. Second, he participated in the International Symposium for Cestode Zoonoses Control, held on 15th–16th, November 2017 in Chengdu, China, with an aim to promote the update and control of echinococcosis and taeniasis/cysticercosis. Due to his active participation of drafting the agenda and invitation of international experts, this meeting was successful with an outcome of what is now referred to as the Chengdu Declaration signed by all participants. Third, his participation in the 27th World Congress of Echinococcosis, held in Algiers, Algeria on 4th–7th October 2017 made an output of an opinion article supported by experts from WHO and National Institute of Parasitic Diseases at China CDC. The article entitled "Combating echinococcosis in China: strengthening the research and development" was published in the journal Infectious Diseases of Poverty. Fourth, his help collecting data on the current status of drug treatment for echinococcosis at the global level, consisted in designing of the questionnaire to collect the information on drug treatment against echinococcosis and collecting the global data on this disease. This internship stimulated his study on control strategy of food-borne parasitic diseases, and pushed his completion of his Ph.D. programme in the field of NTDs.

4.4 Case study 4: Achievements of EQAs on NTDs from 2012 to 2015

NTDs have a significant impact on health and economies throughout the Western Pacific Region. The NIPD, in collaboration with the WPRO, initiated an annual regional EQA for the national reference or public health laboratories in detecting NTD parasitic infections from 2012 to 2015. The goal of the EQA was to assess the performance of the participating laboratories in diagnosing parasites using morphological and serological tests.

Reference or public health laboratories at national level working on NTDs in six countries (Cambodia, China, Lao PDR, Malaysia, Philippines and Vietnam) for the EQAs were preselected by WHO. Two staff of each participating laboratory were invited to NIPD for a two-day assessment. The participants performed serological tests (IHA and ELISA) and helminth morphological microscopy to detect parasitic infections using the same prepared samples. In the serological tests, 20 serum samples were detected by commercial IHA and ELISA kits, while in the morphological tests ten samples of helminth eggs (*Ascaris lumbricoides*, *Clonorchis sinensis*, *Fasciolopsis buski*, *Hookworm*, *Hymenolepis nana*, *Paragonimus westermani*, *Enterobius vermicularis*, *Schistosoma japonicum*, *Spirometra mansoni*, *Taenia* and *Trichuris trichiura*) were diagnosed using Kato-Katz and the direct smear method. The same criteria was used to score the results from each laboratory and the Cut-off point for passing the assessment was set at 60% for the four diagnostic methods used in the assessment. All laboratories consistently scored high in ELISA tests in all 4 years except Lab A in the first EQA. The total coincidence rates of ELISA between 2012 and 2015 were 90%, 99.29%, 94.29% and 98.75%, respectively. For the IHA test, all laboratories passed the test despite one laboratory failed in 2 consecutive years (2013 and 2014). The total coincidence rates of IHA were 100%, 95%, 90% and 97.50% from 2012 to 2015. When the titres of samples were taken into consideration, the coincidence rates for serum samples with titre = 1:20 or 1:10 was lower than those for serum samples with titre = 1:40, especially a very low ratio was recorded in 2013. This result showed that detecting low levels of serum antibody in patients with schistosomiasis remained problematic for the IHA test. The ratio of laboratories which had scored $\geq$60 in different years for direct smear test were 80% (2012), 71.43% (2013), 100% (2014) and 75% (2015), while for the Kato-Katz test were 80% (2012), 57.14% (2013), 100% (2014) and

37.50% (2015), respectively. The overall past rates (score ≥ 60) for direct smear (82.60%) were higher than these for Kato-Katz (68.65%). The detection rate of helminth eggs varied in different species in the direct smear test, with *A. lumbricoides* being the highest at 94.07% in average and *S. mansoni* (29.63%) was lowest. In the Kato-Katz test, the highest rate of detection was negative slide (90.91%) and the lowest was *S. mansoni* (13.64%).

EQA results from 2012 to 2015 indicated that there was an improvement with the laboratories' capacity in diagnosing helminths although some of them still need improvement especially in morphological tests. The detection rates of different species of eggs varied with direct smear test or Kato-Katz test. Some participants could identify the eggs (such as *S. japonicum* eggs, *P. westermani* eggs) using the direct smear method, but could not identify the same eggs using the Kato-Katz method, which means that the participants needed to improve the capacity of discriminating. Another issue was that some laboratories had problems in judging the results obtained from the ELISA or IHA and not highly skilled in serological detection methods. Due to the participants needed more comprehensive coverage of the helminths diagnosis, a training contained the topics of "Serological tests for the detection of *Schistosoma japonicum* infection" and "Helminths egg examination in Stool" was arranged after the EQAs in 2014 and 2015. The training proved to be very useful for the laboratory staff to improve and strengthen their capacity in diagnosing parasitic infections. The EQA programme was a useful way to assess the capacity in helminthiasis diagnosis of participating laboratories and provide opportunities for diagnostic experience sharing. The programme also corrects deficiencies and improve laboratories' proficiency in diagnosing parasitic diseases through training and discussion on the diagnostic tests used in the assessment. NIPD and WPRO aim to continuously conduct the EQA yearly and expand to other laboratories and countries participating in this programme, establish a standardizing network of reference laboratories in detecting NTDs' parasitic infections.

5. Capacity building opportunities

The opportunities of training through the $RNAS^+$ platform is mainly contributed by several host institutions that proactively involved in the $RNAS^+$ activities, including Swiss TPH, Switzerland; QIMR Berghofer, Australia; RITM, the Philippines; UP, the Philippines; NIPD, China; the Veterinary University of Khon Kaen in Thailand; and Louisiana State University in the United States.

5.1 Swiss TPH, Basel, Switzerland

Swiss TPH offers a unique learning experience in a wide range of topics, including international health, epidemiology, public health, infection biology, clinical practice, insurance medicine and management. Three distinct but complementary teaching levels train students from all over the world in these topics. Swiss TPH offers undergraduate and master opportunities, as well as doctoral and Ph.D. programmes in association with the University of Basel. At the postgraduate level, Swiss TPH provides a range of professional certificates (CAS), diplomas (DAS) and master (MAS) programme.

Swiss TPH's unique combination of research, services and training shapes the course curricula and provides participants a multidisciplinary view of the complex interactions between health, diseases and health systems. Novel contributions to science can be introduced and applied in classrooms or through blended learning methods without delay.

Mutual learning is a core principle of Swiss TPH. The professional postgraduate programmes in particular offer lively platforms for exchanging experiences due to the diversity of participants and their professional backgrounds. Swiss TPH engages in joint programmes with global organizations, as well as in national and international education networks and projects, such as the Swiss School of Public Health (SSPH+) and tropEd, the worldwide network for education in international health. Swiss TPH is an associated institute of the University of Basel, the oldest university in Switzerland and internationally known for its outstanding achievements in research and teaching, particularly in life sciences. The close cooperation between the institute and the university enriches the curricula and offers additional study possibilities. The University of Basel provides the official accreditation for all Swiss TPH programmes and courses.

5.2 QIMR Berghofer, Brisbane, Australia

This is one of the largest medical research institutes in Australia with over 750 staff and students. It has a long history in researching tropical medicine and tropical infectious diseases and has been involved in research and research training with $RNAS^+$ since its inception. The research collaborations have been mainly with Khon Kaen University (establishment of field and clinical sites for studying the epidemiology and pathology of opisthorchiasis; training in these areas at QIMR Berghofer and University of Queensland); UP and RITM, the Philippines (involvement in a Tropical Medicine Research

Centre (TMRC) supported by the US National Institutes of Health (NIH) to research and teaching courses on schistosomiasis in the Philippines); and the Chinese Center for Tropical Diseases (CTDR) in Shanghai (the establishment of two TMRCs to research the epidemiology and control of schistosomiasis and hookworm disease and to provide training both in Brisbane and Shanghai in preparing research papers, epidemiological techniques, biostatistics, mathematical modelling, molecular diagnostics, bioinformatics, and data entry processes and data management procedures).

5.3 RITM, Muntinlupa, the Philippines

The RITM Center for Training in Tropical Infectious Diseases was established in 1989, with main function of conducting regular training courses for medical and paramedical personnel in the control of common tropical diseases in the country. RITM provides high quality tertiary care to both in-patients and out-patients suffering from tropical diseases included within the scope of the Institute's research activities.

5.4 NIPD, China CDC, China

This is the sole specialized institution for parasitology at the national level. NIPD is also serving as Chinese Center for Tropical Diseases (CTDR) since 2017. Over the past two decades, sponsored by WHO, other international agencies or bilateral collaborative projects, NIPD has been developed as one of excellency centers for tropical diseases reserach and control. Currently its major tasks are research, training and engaging in global health. In terms of training, NIPD provides degree education and advanced training courses, which includes a Masters degree programme, a Ph.D. programme and postdoctoral fellowships.

The Masters degree programme involves (i) medicine discipline including immunology, pathogenic biology; (ii) public health and preventive medicine including epidemiology and public health statistics; and (iii) master of public health including tropical disease prevention and control. The Ph.D. degree programme and postdoctoral fellowships involve multidisciplinary researches and multisubjects on epidemiology, parasite and vector biology, pathology, immunology, molecular biology, pharmaceutical chemistry and pharmacology. Most of those programmes are focus on research on epidemiological patterns and modelling, transmission features, control strategy and surveillance of malaria, schistosomiasis, filariasis, echinococcosis, kala-azar, soil-transmitted and food-borne parasitic infections.

The advanced training courses are designed to promote the knowledge, skills and capabilities for professionals who conduct research or work in the field. Each year, over 20 workshops and training courses take place in NIPD, most of which sponsored by WHO and the National Health Commission of China. The topics include but not limited to (i) malaria surveillance, forecasting and early warning system; (ii) monitoring of anti-malaria drug's treatment, (iii) medical malacology; (iv) GIS application and modelling in tropical diseases; (v) Global health and tropical diseases; (vi) preparation of scientific papers; and (vii) project management and planning.

NIPD has a strong faculty team, consisting of 6 doctoral supervisors including 2 on epidemiology and health statistics, 2 on immunology, 2 on pathogenic biology; 13 master's tutors including 11 on scientific research, 2 on public health. All researches are supported by the platform named Key Laboratory for Parasitic Pathogens and Vector Biology of National Health Committee. The laboratory not only offers technical team support on stable and high-quality service for equipment use, but also offers the good facility for the research, such as automatic protein purification workstation, biochip spotting instrument, biochip scanner, protein two-dimensional electrophoresis instrument, chip hybridization analyser, ultracentrifuge, gel image analyser and freeze dryer are configured; microplate reader, flow cytometry, chromosomal immunohistochemical analysis system; automatic nucleic acid extraction workstation, DNA sequencer, real-time PCR instrument; laser confocal microscope, biomolecular imager, fluorescence inverted microscope; high performance liquid chromatography, gas chromatography, mass spectrometry, etc.

6. Conclusion

The overall aim of RNAS$^+$ is to strengthen collaboration and control authorities in the endemic countries in the field of zoonotic helminthiasis in Southeast Asia. While sustainable training as capacity building activities has produced great impacts of RNAS$^+$ in terms of strengthening collaboration in multidisciplines, including biology, epidemiology, geographic medicine, ecology, data management, etc. (Bizimana et al., 2018; Dong et al., 2018). With more training activities, more young scientists from the RNAS$^+$ member countries had the trained, but also they started to contribute to the development of RNAS$^+$ by involving the collaborative research projects and participating the discussion in the annual workshop (Liang et al., 2018; Qian et al., 2019). Suggestions from RNAS$^+$-organized

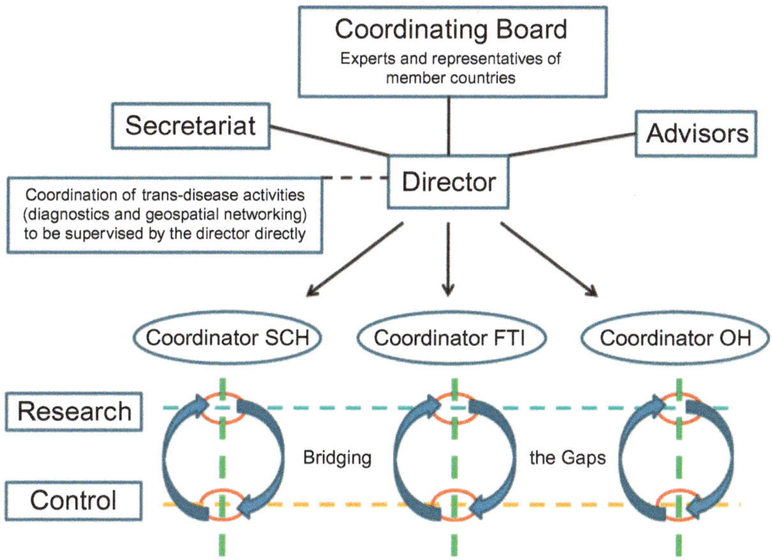

Fig. 1 Schematic functioning of RNAS[+].

workshop discussions, for example, the capacity building need to focus on platform design and technical standardization aiming at fostering research capacity in the future. Moreover, more MOOC projects need to be created under $RNAS^+$ platform which will take the advantages of established networking (Fig. 1). In order to achieve the main goal of $RNAS^+$, the capacity building will certainly be the core activities under $RNAS^+$ platform.

References

Bizimana, P., Polman, K., Van Geertruyden, J.P., Nsabiyumva, F., Ngenzebuhoro, C., Muhimpundu, E., Ortu, G., 2018. Capacity gaps in health facilities for case management of intestinal schistosomiasis and soil-transmitted helminthiasis in Burundi. Infect. Dis. Poverty 7 (1), 66.

Ceccato, P., Ramirez, B., Manyangadze, T., Gwakisa, P., Thomson, M.C., 2018. Data and tools to integrate climate and environmental information into public health. Infect. Dis. Poverty 7 (1), 126.

de Sousa, S.R.M., Dias, I.H.L., Fonseca, A.L.S., Contente, B.R., Nogueira, J.F.C., da Costa Oliveira, T.N., Geiger, S.M., Enk, M.J., 2019. Concordance of the point-of-care circulating cathodic antigen test for the diagnosis of intestinal schistosomiasis in a low endemicity area. Infect. Dis. Poverty 8 (1), 37.

Dong, Y., Du, C.H., Zhang, Y., Wang, L.F., Song, J., Wu, M.S., Yang, W.C., Lv, S., Zhou, X.N., 2018. Role of ecological approaches to eliminating schistosomiasis in Eryuan County evaluated by system modelling. Infect. Dis. Poverty 7 (1), 129.

Liang, S., Abe, E.M., Zhou, X.N., 2018. Integrating ecological approaches to interrupt schistosomiasis transmission: opportunities and challenges. Infect. Dis. Poverty 7 (1), 124.

Lu, Y., Gonzales, G., Chen, S.H., Li, H., Cai, Y.C., Chu, Y.H., Ai, L., Chen, M.X., Chen, H.N., Chen, J.X., 2017. Urgent needs in fostering neglected tropical diseases (NTDs) laboratory capacity in WHO Western Pacific Region: results from the external quality assessment on NTDs diagnosis in 2012–2015. Infect. Dis. Poverty 6 (1), 106.

Olveda, R., Leonardo, L., Zheng, F., Sripa, B., Bergquist, R., Zhou, X.N., 2010. Coordinating research on neglected parasitic diseases in Southeast Asia through networking. Adv. Parasitol. 72, 55–77.

Osorio, L., Garcia, J.A., Parra, L.G., Garcia, V., Torres, L., Degroote, S., Ridde, V., 2018. A scoping review on the field validation and implementation of rapid diagnostic tests for vector-borne and other infectious diseases of poverty in urban areas. Infect. Dis. Poverty 7 (1), 87.

Qian, M.B., Zhou, C.H., Zhu, H.H., Zhu, T.J., Huang, J.L., Chen, Y.D., Zhou, X.N., 2019. Assessment of health education products aimed at controlling and preventing helminthiases in China. Infect. Dis. Poverty 8 (1), 22.

Wang, X.Y., Xu, J., Zhao, S., Li, W., Zhang, J.F., He, J., Swing, A.M., Yang, K., 2018. Estimating the prevalence of schistosomiasis japonica in China: a serological approach. Infect. Dis. Poverty 7 (1), 62.

Yang, X., Zhang, Y., Sun, Q.X., Zhou, J.X., Zhou, X.N., 2019. SWOT analysis on snail control measures applied in the national schistosomiasis control programme in the People's Republic of China. Infect. Dis. Poverty 8 (1), 13.

Zhou, X.N., Olveda, R., Sripa, B., Yang, G.J., Leonardo, L., Bergquist, R., 2015. From gap analysis to solution and action: the $RNAS^+$ model. Acta Trop. 141 (Pt. B), 146–149.

CHAPTER FOUR

From country control programmes to translational research

Lydia Leonardo[a], Robert Bergquist[b], Remigio Olveda[c], Fadjar Satrija[d], Banchob Sripa[e], Somphou Sayasone[f], Virak Khieu[g], Arve Lee Willingham[h], Juerg Utzinger[i], Xiao-Nong Zhou[j,*]

[a]Institute of Biology, College of Science, University of the Philippines Diliman and University of the East Ramon Magsaysay Graduate School, Quezon City, Philippines
[b]Geospatial Health, Ingerod, Brastad, Sweden
[c]Asian Tropical Foundation, Filinvest Corporate City, Research Institute for Tropical Medicine Compound, Muntinlupa, Philippines
[d]Bogor Agricultural University (IPB), JL. Agatis, Kampus IPB, Bogor, Indonesia
[e]Department of Pathology, Khon Kaen University, Khon Kaen, Thailand
[f]Lao Tropical and Public Health Institute, Vientianne, Lao People's Democratic Republic
[g]National Helminth Control Program, National Center for Parasitology, Entomology and Malaria Control Ministry of Health, Phnom Penh, Cambodia
[h]One Health Center for Zoonoses and Tropical Veterinary Medicine, Ross University School of Veterinary Medicine, Basseterre, West Indies
[i]Swiss Tropical and Public Health Institute, Basel, Switzerland
[j]National Institute of Parasitic Diseases, Chinese Center for Disease Control and Prevention; Chinese Center for Tropical Diseases Research; WHO Collaborating Centre for Tropical Diseases, China; National Center for International Research on Tropical Diseases, China; Key Laboratory of Parasite and Vector Biology, Ministry of Health, China, Shanghai, China
*Corresponding author: e-mail address: zhouxn1@chinacdc.cn

Contents

1. Introduction 70
2. Significant developments 71
   2.1 Diagnostics 71
   2.2 Vaccine research 73
   2.3 Drug development 73
3. Database for surveillance in the elimination phase 74
4. New guides for clinicians 78
5. High burdens of target diseases generate interest in control 80
6. Review of control programmes 82
7. Components needed for successful control programmes 84
8. Success stories: Elimination of LF 88
9. Conclusion 89
References 89
Further reading 92

Advances in Parasitology, Volume 105
ISSN 0065-308X
https://doi.org/10.1016/bs.apar.2019.07.005

Abstract

From the time it was conceptualized in 1998 to the present, RNAS$^+$ has largely concentrated on research that will generate results to facilitate control, prevention and elimination of its target diseases. Diagnostics has remained an active field of research in order to develop tools that are appropriate for each stage from the first efforts until attempts to block transmission. For example, with regard to schistosomiasis, chemotherapy has excellent impact on morbidity, while better diagnostics and vaccine research have been promoted to complement the other components of the control programme. The need for surveillance in areas where the prevalence has been brought down to very low levels necessitated development of spatio-temporal tools and ecological models based on geographical information systems (GIS) to produce risk and distribution maps for monitoring and evaluation of programme success. New knowledge and experiences in management of the diseases contribute to the formulation of new schemes in management and treatment. Ways of drawing attention to the disease, such as determining disability weights for use in computation of burden of disease, updating epidemiological profile and unravelling new aspects of the disease provide bases for modifying the operation of control programmes as we move forward. Programme evaluation based on reports of actual implementation of activities brought to the fore problems related to the distribution of chemotherapy as well as social, cultural and behavioural aspects of endemic communities. Importantly, this highlighted the necessity of adapting control activities to specific situations of the endemic areas. New models evolving from reviews of this kind and success stories, such us the elimination of lymphatic filariasis (LF) in PR China and Cambodia are presented.

1. Introduction

Research concentrating on various aspects of the target diseases that will facilitate their control and prevention has always been the focus of the Regional Network on Asian Schistosomiasis and other Helminthic Zoonoses (RNAS$^+$). Annual meetings of the network showcase research findings and advances of member institutions and countries that are expected to address obstacles in control and clarify issues to better implement control programs. As control targets are reached and the disease situation improves considerably, new and more relevant fields emerge such as enhancement of diagnostics, development of surveillance tools and more comprehensive database systems and integration of other disciplines and sectors in the programmes. This chapter presents advances in these fields that are foreseen to untangle current snags in the control, prevention and eventual elimination of RNAS$^+$ target diseases.

2. Significant developments

2.1 Diagnostics

In the early years of RNAS$^+$, Zhu et al. (2002) developed a rapid, simple immunodiagnostic assay for schistosomiasis using soluble egg antigen of *S. japonicum* conjugated with a blue colloidal dye and used to determine antibodies in sera of schistosomiasis patients. Results of field trials show the dipstick dye immunoassay (DDIA) to have high sensitivity and high specificity in detecting schistosomiasis aside from the advantages of being rapid, simple and cheap and without need for special equipment. It was deemed more useful compared to other immunoassays in screening target populations to identify cases for selective chemotherapy. This tool was successfully used in Lao PDR and Cambodia for detection of schistosomiasis mekongi.

Zhang et al. (2016) reviewed the development and use of parasitological, immunodiagnostic and molecular techniques in the diagnosis of schistosomiasis concluding that the main techniques that performed well in the past are not as efficient at present use because of the progress and success in control that have brought prevalence and intensity to levels close to elimination in many areas, in particular in PR China. A flexible approach is recommended to be used in the choice of the most appropriate diagnostic technique relevant for each control stage and area as well as varying the methodology based on the prevailing needs of sensitivity and specificity (Bergquist et al., 2009). Diagnostic tools should be an integral part of the national control programme and should include collaboration among research laboratories, epidemiologists and control programme managers.

Li et al. (2018) presented the evaluation of the performance of four immunodiagnostic kits for detecting clonorchiasis in China in order to address the limitations of other less sensitive techniques. Compliance with respect to submission of stool samples is also low, not to mention the reluctance of health personnel to handle stools. Molecular techniques such as PCR and LAMP may be highly sensitive; however, their cost and high risk with regard to contamination may prevent them from field use. Immunological diagnosis has become the technique of choice especially for its high sensitivity and specificity in low-intensity infections. Results of the evaluation show a relatively high performance of three diagnostic kits in detecting IgG, while the kit for detecting IgM did not perform as well as the former.

The kits that detect IgG show high sensitivity for heavier intensities of infection but is not completely reliable in area characterized by low-intensity of infection, hence the need to improve sensitivity and specificity.

Diagnostic techniques such as examination of stool, urine and biopsy material for the presence of schistosome eggs, detection of antibodies or antigens in patient body fluids and molecular techniques to detect DNA are all limited by their inability to show the severity of end organ pathology and resulting complications due to the lesions. Prolonged and extensive use of antischistosomal drugs such as praziquantel cause changes in the clinical manifestations of the disease. Olveda et al. (2014c) showed advantages in using ultrasonography to assess morbidity in schistosomiasis. The group presented several advantages of ultrasonography over other imaging techniques, such as *computer tomography* (CT) and magnetic resonance imaging (MRI). Ultrasound provides real-time images without acquisition or processing delay; it is not only portable and can be brought to the point of care (POC), but is also cheaper and does not use harmful ionizing radiation. Doppler ultrasound is more advanced providing additional prognostic information aside from the routine grey-scale ultrasound imagery. MRI however can be used in getting into sites that ultrasound may not be able to visualize.

A review done by Olveda et al. (2014a) show that eggs cause bowel lesions ranging from colitis to polyp formation. In the liver, granuloma formation and subsequent fibrosis involve immune responses initially mediated by Th1 and later by Th2 lymphocytes. As a result of severe fibrosis, there may be portal hypertension-related complications causing significant morbidity and eventually death. Liver biopsy and imaging techniques such as ultrasonography, CT and MRI can assess hepatosplenic disease for proper management. There are also new serum markers that are most promising for the evaluation of schistosome-induced hepatic fibrosis, namely, hyaluronic acid, collagen type III, YKL-40 and laminin. Because of the strong correlation between the expression profile of miRNAs and the disease status/progression, circulating host miRNAs can be possibly used biomarkers for schistosomiasis diagnosis. Fabre et al. (2011) suggest that the Tissue Inhibitor of Metalloproteinase-1 (TIMP-1) is a promising biomarker for assessing risk of hepatic fibrosis in schistosomiasis and, potentially, other infectious and non-infectious causes of liver disease. With the use of a multiplex assay that quantifies predictors and effect modifiers of fibrosis (FibroPlex), these authors (2011) show that individuals with detectable tissue inhibitor of TIMP-1 have a 3.5-fold greater risk of fibrosis 1 year after praziquantel treatment. Since TIMP-1 inhibits most enzymes responsible for collagen degradation, the results indicate that schistosome-associated hepatic fibrosis could arise from excessive inhibition of collagen remodelling.

2.2 Vaccine research

The potential of vaccine development continues to be explored especially with mathematical models showing the effective contribution of a vaccine when added to the conventional components of the control programme. Shi et al. (2002) developed two experimental DNA vaccines that have been proved to be capable of inducing protection in water buffalos that are naturally exposed to schistosome infection in the field. In the field trial of the vaccines in cattle, worm and egg counts conducted at the end of the experiment showed partial resistance in each vaccine group. It is envisioned that these vaccines would be combined with selective population chemotherapy of both human and bovine populations. The group evaluation vaccines recommended more trials to determine whether protection can be improved with vaccination of multiple DNA plasmids compared to single administration of individual DNA vaccines.

Jiz et al. (2008) developed a pilot scale expression and purification scheme for recombinant full-length *S. japonicum* paramyosin, while Wu et al. (2017) in a follow-up study conducted three vaccine trials to assess the efficacy of recombinant full-length paramyosin (rSj 97) in protecting water buffalos from infection. Lower worm burdens were recorded for buffalos immunized with the recombinant molecule indicating that rSj97 is a safe and promising molecule for use as vaccine against schistosomiasis japonica in water buffalos.

2.3 Drug development

Pakharukova et al. (2015) conducted the first functional study of the flatworm cytochrome P450 (CYP) enzyme in *Opisthorchis felineus*, which causes biliary tract diseases in Russia, Kazakhstan and central Europe. This enzyme belongs to a group of proteins that are specifically involved in the synthesis of physiologically active compounds, in drug metabolism, and in biotransformation of xenobiotics. Although only one CYP450 enzyme was identified in *O. felineus*, this could be a promising drug target but a better understanding the physiology of this liver fluke is needed before a drug can be developed.

Jiang et al. (2017) developed an *in situ* slow-release formulation of praziquantel by subcutaneous injection, which should be capable of resisting new *Echinococcus* infections for at least 6 months.

Jia et al. (2019) reported a new compound Luo-Wei from the plant extracts against the intermediate host snails in China and Egypt, and evaluate its environmental safety to non-target organisms. It was demonstrated that this drug was active against *O. hupensis*, *B. alexandrina* and *B. truncatus* under laboratory and field conditions, and it may be a candidate molluscicide of plant origin.

3. Database for surveillance in the elimination phase

The relevance and success of control programmes depend on the initial data used in developing the various strategies to be implemented. As targets are achieved and prevalence goes down, surveillance becomes a necessity in following up and treating the remaining infected humans and reservoirs and monitoring intermediate hosts and environmental conditions that perpetuate infections.

Distribution of opisthorchiasis viverrini includes Thailand, Lao PDR and Cambodia where the disease is considered a major public health problem. To ascertain the extent and distribution of opisthorchiasis in Cambodia, Miyamoto et al. (2014) conducted surveys that found four Cambodian provinces to be endemic to the disease. The group proposed a more widespread nationwide survey to complement the partial results obtained. Furthermore, they recommended that field surveys be carefully planned to address the complex environmental factors that could influence distribution of *O. viverrini* infections in endemic areas.

Sithithaworn et al. (2012) assessed the present situation and control of liver fluke infections such as *O. viverrini* and *Clonorchis sinensis* in the Mekong Basin countries. Most recent data on prevalence and distribution were obtained from presentations during the "96 Years of Opisthorchiasis. International Congress of Liver Flukes" held in Khon Kaen, Thailand on March 7–8, 2011.They found that in spite of treatment and control programmes enforced for decades, the two liver flukes remain in high prevalence in all countries of the Lower Mekong Basin with the situation aggravated by the frighteningly high levels of the circulating cathodic antigen (CCA). It was noted that in each endemic country there is higher transmission in the lowlands resulting in higher prevalence compared with that in the highlands. The high transmission in the lowlands has been correlated with wetlands, flooding patterns and more human movement and settlements.

Qian and Zhou (2017) reported that scarce and deficient data coupled with the complex and chronic nature of cancers make it difficult to obtain a correct valuation of how many cases of cholangiocarcinoma can be associated with liver flukes. Research should be intensified to obtain correct data which could be used to raise awareness of the impact of liver flukes in east Asia and hence advance control and prevention strategies.

Angiostrongyliasis caused by the nematode *Angiostrongylus cantonensis* is a food borne-parasitic zoonosis transmitted by consumption of molluscs infected with the third stage larvae of the parasite. Hu et al. (2018) investigated the infection status and spatial distribution of the rodent and mollusc host in three villages from Nanao Island in Guangdong Province, PR China which could be used as basis in developing appropriate strategy for prevention and control of the disease. Results showed positive spatial correlation in the distribution of the mollusc host *Pomacea canaliculata* and rats. It was concluded that there is a risk of angiostrongyliasis in the island and therefore both mollusc and rodent hosts should be intensely monitored.

Li et al. (2007) concluded that three approaches that were adopted to accurately describe the epidemiology of schistosomiasis in PR China were national sampling survey, active sentinel surveillance and passive routine report. Results from these methods showed an increase in schistosomiasis which was attributed to a better reporting system rather than real increase in incidence. The integrated control strategy in 2004 brought down the prevalence of schistosomiasis considerably spurring PR China to aim for elimination by 2025.

PR China is known for its high endemicity for echinococcosis that has been given high priority especially in western endemic areas where considerable control activities are being implemented. Recognizing the importance of using dependable data to control the disease, China conducted the largest epidemiological survey from 2012 to 2016 covering all nine endemic provinces. Results revealed the presence of cystic echinococcosis in 368 counties, 115 of which were also co-endemic for alveolar echinococcosis. The necessity for a global database for echinococcosis has been similarly recognized to intensify the fight against this disease. In the late 2017, a network was established in Chengdu, PR China to build capacity for the research and development necessary to reach the control targets for echinococcosis.

Taenia solium has also been selected for strong control activities due to its role in the development of cysticercosis in humans. It is expected that through commitment, coordination and cooperation of all endemic countries and the international community, this infection would be brought under control by 2030. Called the Belt and Road Network for the Elimination and Control of echinococcosis and cysticercosis (B&R-NEC), experts from 13 countries signed the Chengdu Declaration and the network was opened to all countries willing to join the fight against the disease (Qian and Zhou, 2018).

Fasciola hepatica and *F. gigantica* are common parasites among ruminants all over the world causing death among this livestock. Chen et al. (2013) reported an outbreak of human fascioliasis in Yunnan Province caused by consumption of the herb (*Houttuynia cordata*) which local people consume frequently in the summer (June to September). This has been recognized as a new source of infection for fascioliasis in PR China. The group expect that this new information can be integrated into the One Health approach to lessen transmission and virulence of both human and animal fascioliasis. Important intervention measures that should be sustained include health education and cessation of use of animal faeces as fertilizers.

In PR China, two of the most important natural hosts for *S. japonicum* are 'yellow cattle' and water buffalo with the former observed to be more compatible for development of the parasite. Yang et al. (2012a,b) determined the immunological basis for this higher susceptibility of yellow cattle and the more serious pathology that is observed with the infection. This information will certainly be critical in designing vaccines in addition to understanding the mechanism of self-cure in water buffalos that can further advance schistosome vaccine research and application.

Habib et al. (2018) using both morphological and molecular evidences reported that the *Biomphalaria* populations from Guangdong are *B. straminea*, the intermediate host of *S. mansoni* in Brazil. These snails could have been introduced via passive dispersal or through several introduction routes from this country. In the light of increasing reports of active *S. mansoni* infections among workers returning from Africa, increased surveillance for all entry ports and inspection of exotic species are recommended to decrease probability of further introduction of such type of species and emergence of new diseases in PR China.

The study of Yang et al. (2013b) showed the usefulness of spatio-temporal analysis in evaluating the risk for schistosomiasis. Results of mouse bioassay from 2009 to 2011 analysed by directional distributional analysis and scan statistics were used to illustrate the spatio-temporal risk pattern. The spatial distribution was focused along the Yangtze River and the directional distributions for the percentage of infected mice and average worm burdens resemble those observed for positive sentinel sites. The group concluded that this approach would be valuable for surveillance and response especially as progress is achieved in moving from morbidity control to transmission control.

The feasibility of stopping transmission of STH from a global view was considered by Brooker and colleagues and they included China as one of the most feasible groups that can achieve this. The far-reaching economic development and intense helminth control programs of China have greatly impacted control efforts and resulted in the tremendous reduction in soil-transmitted helminth in PR China as shown by the considerable decline in the number of infected people from 536 million in 1988–1992 to 129 million in 2001–2004 and the decreasing trend has since been sustained. Qian et al. (2015) proposed that prevalence and intensity levels reflected at the provincial level could be used as assessment map by policy makers to evaluate progress of interruption of transmission and prioritize provinces for more intensified control measures. General prevalence surveys should be followed by setting up of surveillance spots that will regularly provide real time data to determine progress in transmission interruption in order to adjust the interventions accordingly. The success of transmission interruption in China will not only benefit local people but could create a large impact on worldwide efforts to control STH.

Zhou et al. (2009) reported on the proceedings of the 1st International Symposium on Geospatial Health presentations showed proofs of the wide and extensive use of spatially-explicit analyses and other geospatial approaches across Southeast Asia. Applications of these approaches on parasitic infections with considerable impact in the region such as soil-transmitted, food-borne and water-borne helminthic infections, lymphatic filariasis (LF), leishmaniasis and malaria were shown. Advances in GIS and satellite-generated remote-sensing techniques together with spatial statistics have been utilized to show the impact of climate change and ecological transformations.

Examples of these include time series analyses, advanced modelling and Bayesian geostatistics in addition to random-effect models and transmission dynamics can improve knowledge about epidemiology of schistosomiasis and control. Geospatial tools are expected to provide warnings especially in areas further north where schistosomiasis is expected to advance as a consequence of climate change. The spread of disease as a consequence of large-scale water resources development and management projects such as the Three Gorges Dam completed in 2009 and the South-North Water Transfer Project under construction currently can be effectively monitored through these advanced geo-spatial tools (Yang et al., 2013a).

The symposium showed current initiatives that prove that remotely-sensed environmental data and advanced mathematical modelling in a spatially-explicit framework can be used to monitor demographic, eco-epidemiological and socio-economic changes and from these develop early warning systems to mitigate possible detrimental consequences of climate change or other massive and drastic ecological changes. Applications are not only limited to human public health but extended to veterinary medicine.

Schistosomiasis is still endemic in 7 out of the 12 original endemic provinces in PR China. The control of the snail intermediate host *Oncomelania hupensis* is crucial in the elimination of the disease. However, schistosomiasis endemic areas in hilly and mountainous areas in China are much more complicated and difficult to access making efficient and accurate snail surveys extremely hard to conduct compared to the endemic areas located in plains/swamp and lake regions.

Zhu et al. (2015) proposed an ecological niche model integrated with NDVI, LST, elevation, slope and distance from every village to its nearest stream that has satisfactorily predicted the snail habitats in the mountainous region. The model was validated in two counties with the same ecological conditions in Yunnan Province, PR China producing a predictive value of 76.67% and 83.3% for the two villages. It was concluded that the potential of this model for use in snail surveillance in mountainous regions is high.

In the light of the near elimination status of schistosomiasis in PR China, there is a growing need for a rapid and sensitive technique for monitoring the distribution of infected *O. hupensis* in the remaining endemic areas in the seven endemic provinces. Tong et al. (2015) used LAMP assay targeting 28 SrDNA for the quick and accurate detection of *Schistosoma japonicum* DNA in infected and prepatent infected snails. For the first time, infected snails from field sites of low endemicity areas were successfully monitored by LAMP assay using pooled samples which essentially provides an alternative but a more efficient way of screening of increasing large numbers of samples collected from endemic areas especially those with low endemicity requiring larger number of samples to be collected. The risk map that can be generated from the LAMP results has huge potential in being used as an innovative tool to direct surveillance and response strategies in risk areas that can eventually lead to elimination of the disease in such low endemicity areas (Tong et al., 2015).

4. New guides for clinicians

The study of Olveda et al. (2017) showed that treatment with praziquantel produced a short-term impact on prevalence and intensity of infection but little impact on morbidity that has already set in. The grade of liver fibrosis was found to be associated with higher tissue inhibitor of TIMP-1 and hyaluronic acid serum levels and enhanced liver fibrosis (ELF) cut-off score of 8. These figures therefore can be used by physicians in identifying individuals who are more predisposed to serious morbidity. Programme managers can therefore be guided in allocating their resources to areas where they are needed. In addition, the ELF test could be made available and affordable in the field for use by clinicians to evaluate patients with heavy intensities of infection (>400epg) and or those with manifestations of advanced disease (e.g. MCL > 3) to detect their risk of developing severe liver fibrosis.

Olveda et al. (2014b) presented the results of a successful clinical management of a 12-year-old boy in the advanced stage of schistosomiasis from the province of Northern Samar, the Philippines. Massive bleeding due to ruptured oesophageal varices and pancytopenia due to hypersplenism are the major complications of portal hypertension in schistosomiasis with massive bleeding causing majority of the deaths from the disease. The group proposed that for bleeding oesophageal or gastric varices, the best immediate procedure is endoscopy-guided injection sclerotherapy or band ligation of the bleeding varices. The group recognized the limitation in facilities and expertise in developing countries and recommended vasoactive drugs to lower the splanchnic vascular pressure as a temporary solution. As was done in the reported patient, splenectomy is recommended as an appropriate and possibly life-saving procedure for patients with considerably large spleens with pancytopenia caused by hypersplenism but with no history of bleeding from oesophageal or gastric varices and without ascites.

Sripa et al. (2017) reviewed most recent results that deal with the role played by liver-fluke associated *Helicobacter pylori* in hepatobiliary disease and malignancy. The group proposed that the presence of both *O. viverrini* and *H. pylori* is at the core of liver fluke infection associated with cholangiocarcinoma. Recent literature point to liver fluke being a reservoir of *Helicobacter* spp. and explains the role of liver fluke associated *H. pylori* in hepatobiliary disease and malignancy.

Gouveia et al. (2017) report results that show that *O. felineus* should be included in the Group 1 list of biological carcinogens just like its related flukes *O. viverrini* and *C. sinensis*. Biochemical and histopathological changes resulting from *O. felineus* infection in the rodent model led to formation of precancerous lesions contributing to malignancy.

Coutinho et al. (2005) concludes that, in children, adolescents, and young adults infected with *S. japonicum*, hepatic fibrosis is associated with impaired nutritional status. Early recognition and treatment of this type of morbidity can be critical because of the strong evidence linking malnutrition with the detrimental effects on morbidity, mortality, cognitive development, reproduction, and the capacity for physical activity. The group further show that even low-grade hepatic fibrosis is associated with significantly worse nutritional status. These researchers hypothesized that it could lead to malnutrition and anaemia through a systemic increase in the levels of proinflammatory cytokines, specifically IL-1 and IL-6, and possibly TNF-α.

Wieringa et al. (2016) conducted a national micronutrient survey in children and women that was linked to the Cambodian Demographic Health Survey 2014 (CDHS-2014) to determine the prevalence of micronutrient deficiency, haemoglobin disorders and intestinal parasite infection. Results of the survey were meant to provide data on causes of anaemia which is a condition highly prevalent among Cambodian women and children with over 50% under 5-year old suffering from the condition. The survey revealed that the very high prevalence of anaemia in Cambodian women and children cannot be attributed solely to micronutrient deficiencies and haemoglobin disorders. Therefore, micronutrient interventions to reduce anaemia prevalence would possibly have limited impact in the Cambodian setting. Iron deficiency prevalence was found to be low in children above 2 years of age and in women. Wieringa et al. (2016) recommended that the focus of the present interventions to decrease the high prevalence of anaemia in children and women should be expanded and should involve provision of zinc and folic acid for women of reproductive age, as well as effective anti-hookworm measures.

5. High burdens of target diseases generate interest in control

Clonorchiasis is a recognized public health problem in PR China. However, Qian et al. (2013b) noted that researches are not enough to generate needed information of the disease. The group suggested that the serious threat of clonorchiasis to public health in PR China can be demonstrated by comparing this disease with hepatitis B in terms of epidemiology, clinical symptoms and carcinogenicity, disability and changing trends. It is expected that the intensity of control efforts put forth by PR China will impact considerably on the global agenda for control and elimination of this disease.

More researches are therefore awaited from Chinese researchers which hopefully will snowball and expand to include international cooperation.

Paragonimiasis, caused by the lung fluke *Paragonimus* spp., is a food-borne trematodiasis (FBT) and one of the 20 NTDs on the WHO list. The suffering caused by this disease is however not that well understood. In addition, quantification by the disability weight of the DALYs is largely variable in various global burden of disease (GBD) estimates. The top two contributors to disability weight are lung outcomes and headache. Feng et al. (2018) conclude from the systematic analysis that they did that further modification should be done to calculate the disease burden of paragonimiasis. This is important for public health prioritization of paragonimiasis in research, monitoring and control.

Torgerson et al. (2015) reported on the initial estimations of 10 helminth diseases and toxoplasmosis that may be associated with contaminated food which could provide deeper understanding of the big effect of food-borne diseases regionally and globally. It was revealed that the disease burden attributed to most food-borne parasites is very focal and leads to substantial morbidity and mortality among vulnerable population groups.

In spite of the impact of clonorchiasis in Southeast Asia and its classification as a biologic carcinogen, it remains unlisted among the Global Burden of Disease (GBD) and disability weight is still lacking. Disability weight refers to the average degree of loss of life value due to a certain chronic condition and ranges between 0 for complete health and 1 for death. It is a very important parameter for estimating the morbidity part of any disease burden in terms of DALYs. Qian et al. (2011) reported the results of their study which was the first attempt to calculate the disability due to clonorchiasis which refers to average loss of life caused by some conditions and crucial for computing for disease burden as expressed as DALYs. The group showed that the overall disability was higher in male compared to female and that there is positive correlation between disability and infection intensity and gallstone got the major attributable proportion. Results may spur further studies that can produce results that can be used for the final estimation of disease burden which in turn can be provide sufficient basis for promoting health awareness and implementation of intervention.

With the recognition of *O. viverrini* as a carcinogenic parasite and the major risk factor for CCA, both government and public sectors have provided more attention to liver fluke surveillance and control. In north-eastern Thailand, for example, academic researchers and public health workers have bonded together for more intense and comprehensive investigations not only of the prevalence of infection but importantly treatment and surgical therapy of CCA. All these concerted efforts are expected to alleviate the situation of the poor suffering from this fatal disease and more successful prevention and control resulting in improved quality of life and increased productivity leading to socioeconomic advances.

Nowadays, the importance of echinococcosis has been demonstrated in China. Many surveys showed the high endemic areas, especially in western areas.

6. Review of control programmes

Chen et al. (2018) presented the 60-year history of schistosomiasis control and prevention in China that reaped considerable success in bringing down levels of the disease to near elimination levels in many endemic areas. Chairman Mao Zedong himself led the intensive campaign calling for elimination of schistosomiasis recognizing the magnitude of the problem in 12 provinces along the Yangtze River. Yujiang County responded immediately and using a multipronged approach composed of snail control through environmental modification, repeated screening and molluscicide treatment for 2 years eventually declared elimination of the disease.

Strong political leadership and support at the highest level of the government have always marked the programme in all three stages of implementation marked by mass campaigns and vertical control focusing on snail eradication in the first stage followed by praziquantel-based morbidity control in the second stage and accelerated implementation of an integrated strategy concentrating on all sources of transmission together with continued snail control, agricultural mechanization construction of lavatories with continuous supply of water and treatment and health education in the third and final stage. Out of the previously 12 endemic provinces, five have eliminated schistosomiasis; one has achieved transmission control and six have reached status of transmission interruption. PR China also helps other endemic countries as shown by the China-Zanzibar-WHO project which also adopted the strategy of high-level government communication and technical cooperation. The importance of socio-economic development in schistosomiasis elimination is seriously recognized and addressed through the current Belt and Road initiative project that is intended to uplift local economies together with global health development.

Xu et al. (2015) reviewed the progress of control programs for major helminthiases in PR China such as schistosomiasis, STH, clonorchiasis and echinococcosis each in a different control stage that requires specific approach. It was concluded that the significant economic development in PR China coupled with the improved consciousness on the burden of parasitic diseases brought about greater attention to control of parasitic diseases. Scientific control policies and control approaches consider different eco-epidemiological settings in their implementation which are expected to eventually succeed in achieving targets for control.

Sustainable financial resources and political commitments can further sustain progress and assure attainment of goals for control, prevention and eventually elimination. Integration of preventive chemotherapy of the different helminthiases requiring broad spectrum anthelminth drugs, such as praziquantel, mebendazole and albendazole is highly possible since endemic areas for these diseases overlap and they are co-endemic with each other. Finally, gains from these efforts can further be magnified to achieve the long term goal of interruption of transmission by improvement of hygiene, housing and sanitation conditions. Provision of safe water supply and latrines for adequate disposal of excreta and solid waste and environmental modification to improve sanitation can decrease contamination of the environment with helminth eggs and reduce transmission of helminthiases.

Progress can be further accelerated through stronger collaboration among different departments like Water Conservancy, Agriculture, Husbandry, and Education. In spite of progress in control, there are still obstacles that have to be overcome to control morbidity and eliminate helminthiases. In 2012, a gap analysis on helminth control was conducted by the diseases reference group on helminth infections (DRG4), a group established in 2009 by the Special Programme for Research and Training in Tropical Diseases (TDR). A research and development agenda for helminthiases control was also promoted covering seven topics such as interventions, diagnostics, basic biology, mathematical modelling, social, and environmental determinants and capacity building. The need for sustainable and additional funding to support more advanced studies is continuously reiterated as well as translation of potential scientific advancements into improved or novel interventions.

Olveda et al. (2014d) concluded that in the Philippines, MDA alone will not be able to control incidence, prevalence and morbidity due to schistosomiasis. The zoonotic nature of the disease where livestock like water buffalos and cattle contribute considerably to the transmission can confound control efforts that are based mainly on MDA. The success of Japan in eliminating schistosomiasis in the 1990s and of China in purging the disease in 5 out of 12 endemic provinces is founded on integrated strategies of snail control, mass chemotherapy of the endemic population, health education, provision of sanitary facilities, environmental modification and improved agricultural methods. Such success may not be expected easily from the Philippines because of the year-round transmission of the disease in the Philippines compared to just 5 months in China in addition to the limited budget allocated for schistosomiasis control. The group proposed that should bovine vaccine be successful in the pilot study that they are conducting, this could be incorporated to an integrated approach composed of human mass chemotherapy, targeted molluscicides and bovine (water buffalo and cattle) treatment.

The cornerstone of the national control programme for schistosomiasis in the Philippines is annual MDA with 40 mg/kg of praziquantel in endemic areas with prevalence of 10% or more. Ross et al. (2015) however concluded that MDA is not enough to control the prevalence and intensity of infection or morbidity of the disease. MDA is marked by increasing problems of inadequate drug coverage, low cure rates, poor drug compliance, absence of baseline information before starting MDA, and insufficient monitoring and evaluation from the time started all of which should be addressed in control programs based on MDA. Multisectoral and intersectorial strategies to complement MDA are clearly needed for more effective control and prevention of the disease.

Collaboration among the community, educational, public health and government sectors is needed to successfully control the disease. The most possible reason for the failure of the control programs could be the paucity of culturally sensitive and proper and clear information about "raw attitudes" in eating behaviour of the people in the Lower Mekong Basin (Ziegler et al., 2013).

7. Components needed for successful control programmes

O. viverrini is one of three very important species of liver flukes that are highly pathogenic to humans and are transmitted by consumption of poorly cooked or raw infected fish. Opisthorchiasis viverrini is an important public health problem in Southeast Asia particularly in Thailand where the prevalence remains high in the north-eastern provinces in spite of the long history of control. Sripa et al. (2015) reported on a new control strategy that he and his group developed called the Lawa model which was introduced in the Lawa Lake area in Khon Kaen province where the liver fluke is highly endemic.

Based on the EcoHealth/One Health Approach, the components of the novel programme included anthelminth treatment, novel intensive health education methods both in the communities and in schools, ecosystem monitoring and active community participation. The new programme resulted in the decrease in infection rate in the 10 villages located around the lake by one-third of the average of 50% from the baseline survey. Infection in the cyprinoid intermediate fish host also went down to 1% compared to the very high 70% baseline prevalence. The Lawa model is presently recognized not only nationally but also internationally as an effective control programme and is being extended to other parts of Thailand and neighbouring Mekong countries. Prior to the development of the Lawa model, community-based surveillance and intervention against FBTs were lacking, particularly with regard to opisthorchiasis.

The current Lawa model is an ecosystem approach to health and is described as transdisciplinary, participatory and considers gender and equity and ecological principals in the development of intervention measures. Variables that are responsible for transmission are identified so that an integrated intervention programme can be developed that has a high degree of sustainability. The Lawa model implemented in villages around the Lawa Lake uses the EcoHealth approach and has been successful in bringing down the prevalence of opisthorchiasis dramatically. A similar strategy called Pilot EcoHealth for human liver fluke was intended for implementation in endemic areas of Lao PDR, Cambodia, Vietnam and southern China.

The success of an intervention programme for schistosomiasis depends on consideration of the socio-ecological context. The eco-social factors influencing existence of perpetuation of schistosomiasis are not that well understood especially at the household or village levels. The study of Yang et al. (2014) showed that the important factors identified in 26 villages of Eryuan county, Yunnan Province, People's Republic of China that are associated with schistosomiasis are absence of a sanitary stall house for livestock and presence of living and infected intermediate host snails in close proximity. The group concluded that an approach involving spatially explicit Bayesian multilevel analysis can help understand more deeply the eco-social determinants that influence schistosomiasis transmission at a small geographical scale.

In PR China, schistosomiasis remains in five provinces of lake and marshland regions and in two provinces mainly composed of mountainous regions. Previous studies have shown that perception both at the individual and community levels, attitudes towards schistosomiasis, and hygiene behaviours are critical factors that influence control and prevention of schistosomiasis. The study of Liu et al. (2014) assessed the knowledge of, attitudes towards, and practices (KAP) relating to schistosomiasis in two subtypes of a mountainous region in Eryuan County, Yunnan Province, PR China. While the overall knowledge rate of schistosomiasis was found to be high in Eryan County, the group recommended that in the light of varying risk factors, control strategies should be crafted in such a way that the different subtypes of endemic areas, namely, plateau basins and plateau canyons for this mountainous region will be carefully considered. For example, consideration should be made of the higher number of risk factors in plateau canyon regions such as frequently grazing cattle, digging vegetables and cutting grass in the field, as well as raising cattle by free grazing compared with the plateau basin regions.

Qian et al. (2013a) proposed the adoption of different intervention measures in different populations because of the varying knowledge, behaviour and infection intensity among population groups. For adults, especially adult males, priority should be given to chemotherapy. Health education particularly focusing on children can eventually yield good results in the long term control of the disease. Restaurants should also be included in the intervention program.

Hung et al. (2015), in a cross-sectional study conducted in Gia Minh and Gia Thinh communes of Gia Vien District, Ninh Binh province found that these communes remain endemic for FBT even if people are aware of the risks of eating raw fish. The group recommended that for a strategy for controlling helminth diseases to succeed, there should be intensified efforts to educate people on the harm due to FBT and the importance of stopping the habit of consumption of raw fish.

Yang et al. (2013b) reviewed emerging and re-emerging diseases that are presently endemic in China such as schistosomiasis, dengue, avian influenza, angiostrongyliasis and soil-transmitted helminthiasis which are concluded to be attributed to environmental and agricultural change. The review reiterated that environmental changes, agricultural practices and social status significantly influence the existing vicious cycle between poverty and infectious diseases. In order to determine the multiple risk factors associated with global changes the following four-pronged approach was recommended by the group composed of the following: identifying metrics, defining risk factors quantitatively and qualitatively, establishment of risk-factor models, and designing policies and programmes for specific disease for decision makers. Assessment plays a critical role in development of intervention strategies that are suited to the local settings and needs to minimize the impact of global change.

In PR China, the application of chemical molluscicides remains as one of the most effective measures for schistosomiasis control. Yang et al. (2012a) investigated the cost-effectiveness of molluscicide application in order to so recommend an optimal management approach to control intermediate host snail *O. hupensis* under acceptable thresholds based on the goal of the National Schistosomiasis Control Programme. The study concluded that different stages of the national schistosomiasis control/elimination programme, namely, morbidity control, transmission control and transmission interruption, should utilize different molluscicide treatment strategies to maximize cost-effectiveness. The group recommended the use of molluscicide treatment once a year to transition from morbidity control to transmission control. Further, environmental modification of snail habitats could be done as an ultimate option during the transition stage from transmission control to transmission interruption. During the stage of post-elimination/transmission interruption, re-emerging snail habitats must be eliminated immediately.

Developing countries have been plagued by tropical diseases which have been a principal cause of morbidity and mortality. Over the past 20 years, collective efforts have been successful in improving the situation but poor communities continue to struggle with these diseases. In general the trend has been declining especially brought about by improvement in the responses to basic health problems and improving health delivery system to vulnerable populations. Based on the WHO's NTD roadmap, the London Declaration on Neglected Tropical Diseases (NTDs) created the direction for control and eventual elimination of several tropical diseases by 2020, giving the thrust for local and regional disease elimination programmes.

In response, the 'First Forum on Surveillance-Response System Leading to Tropical Diseases Elimination' was organized in Shanghai in June 2012 for the purpose of identifying and prioritizing strategic research on elimination of tropical diseases. During the meeting, there was an evaluation of current strategies and the NTD roadmap which was followed by discussions to identify and analyse prevailing challenges and opportunities together with inter-sectoral collaboration and approaches for elimination of several infectious, tropical diseases. The first forum also saw the development of a priority research agenda within a 'One Health-One World' frame of global health. The components of the research agenda included (i) the establishment of a platform for resource-sharing and effective surveillance-response systems for Asia Pacific and Africa with an initial focus on elimination of lymphatic filariasis, malaria and schistosomiasis; (ii) development of new strategies, tools and approaches, such as improved diagnostics and antimalarial therapies; (iii) rigorous validation of surveillance-response systems; and (iv) designing pilot studies to transfer Chinese experiences of successful surveillance-response systems to endemic countries with limited resources.

8. Success stories: Elimination of LF

LF caused by the filarial worms *Wuchereria bancrofti, Brugia malayi* and *B. timori* is a NTD that is a major public health problem in many tropical and subtropical countries. The WHO has targeted the disease for elimination as a public health problem by 2020. The Global Programme to Eliminate LF (GPELF) was established in 2000 based on two very important pillars which are (a) transmission interruption through MDA of antifilarial drugs, and (b) alleviation of suffering in chronic patients through morbidity management and disease prevention (MMDP). Before 2000, LF was endemic in 80 countries where 1.1 billion people are residing in known endemic areas and 120 million people were actually infected. Encouraging advances however such as development of new treatment strategies and introduction of new diagnostic tools in the 1980s and 1990s spurred the WHO to endeavour for global elimination.

Khieu et al. (2018) reported the success of Cambodia in having eliminated LF as a public health problem as validated by WHO in 2016. As one of the first countries in the world to craft and implement an LF elimination program, Cambodia's intense efforts as documented in a dossier submitted to WHO included LF mapping in the country to determine endemic provinces, robust implementation of MDA, regular data collection from sentinel and spot check sites, results from surveys where MDA has been stopped and a summary of post-MDA surveillance activities (TASs 2 and 3). The report also documented how access to chronic LF cases was achieved and how the health system has been training, treating, and monitoring those cases to make sure they get the care they need. In 2015, the Ministry of Health (MoH) of Cambodia put together its final report documenting the elimination of LF as a public health problem and submitted to and validated by the Regional Dossier Review Group of WHO's Western Pacific Regional Office. The following year in June 2016, the WHO headquarters publicly and formally recognized that elimination of LF as a public health problem was achieved in Cambodia.

In PR China, LF was eliminated much earlier in 2006 after decades of sustained efforts focused on multisectoral collaboration involving various departments of the government, intensified control, prevention and elimination programme for LF and continued and massive cooperation from endemic populations (De-jian et al., 2013).

9. Conclusion

The expanded membership of the RNAS$^+$ and the inclusion of other target diseases like other helminthic zoonoses and NTDs endemic in the member countries succeeded in securing attention for majority of parasitic diseases causing public health problems in the Asian region. With prevalence going down and reaching near elimination levels, more sensitive diagnostics are developed and surveillance tools particularly based on spatio-temporal analysis see greater promise in monitoring progress in endemic areas. New disciplines and more sectors are integrated to ensure that all aspects of the disease are considered and addressed. Success in the elimination of LF in Cambodia and China illustrates the magnitude of work involved but also heightens optimism that the goal can be achieved.

References

Bergquist, R., Johansen, M.V., Utzinger, J., 2009. Diagnostic dilemmas in helminthology: what tools to use and when? Trends Parasitol. 25 (4), 151–156. https://doi.org/10.1016/j.pt.2009.01.004.

Chen, J.-X., Chen, M.-X., Ai, L., Xu, X.-N., Jiao, J.-M., Zhu, T.-J., Su, H.-Y., Zang, W., Luo, J.-J., Guo, Y.-H., Lv, S., Zhou, X.-N., 2013. An outbreak of human fascioliasis gigantica in Southwest China. PLoS One 8 (8), e71520. https://doi.org/10.1371/journal.pone.0071520.

Chen, J., Jing, X., Bergquist, R., Li, S.-Z., Zhou, X.-N., 2018. "Farewell to the god of plague": the importance of political commitment towards the elimination of schistosomiasis. Trop. Med. Infect. Dis. 3, 108. https://doi.org/10.3390/tropicalmed3040108.

Coutinho, H.M., McGarvey, S.T., Acosta, L.P., Manalo, D.L., Langdon, G.C., Leenstra, T., Kanzaria, H.K., Solomon, J., Wu, H., Olveda, R.M., Kurtis, J.D., Friedman, J.F., 2005. Nutritional status and serum cytokine profiles in children, adolescents, and young adults with *Schistosoma japonicum*-associated hepatic fibrosis, in Leyte, Philippines. J. Infect. Dis. 192 (3), 528–536.

De-Jian, S., Xu-Li, D., Ji-Hui, D., 2013. The history of the elimination of lymphatic filariasis in China. Infect. Dis. Poverty 2, 30. https://doi.org/10.1186/2049-9957-2-30.

Fabre, V., Wu, H., PondTor, S., Coutinho, H., Acosta, L., Jiz, M., Olveda, R., Cheng, L., White, E.S., Jarilla, B., McGarvey, S.T., Friedman, J.F., Kurtis, J.D., 2011. Tissue inhibitor of matrix-metalloproteasep-1 predicts risk of hepatic fibrosis in human *Schistosoma japonicum* infection. J. Infect. Dis. 203, 707–714.

Feng, Y., Fürst, T., Liu, L., Yang, G.-J., 2018. Estimation of disability weight for paragonimiasis: a systematic analysis. Infect. Dis. Poverty 7, 110.

Gouveia, M.J.o., Maria, Y.P., Laha, T., Sripa, B., Galina, A.M., Rinaldi, G., Paul, J.B., Mordvinov, V.A., Amaro, T., Santos, L.L., da Costa, J.M.C., Vale, N., 2017. Infection with *Opisthorchis felineus* induces intraepithelial neoplasia of the biliary tract in a rodent model. Carcinogenesis 38 (9), 929–937.

Habib, M.R., Lv, S., Guo, Y.-H., Gu, W.-B., Standley, C.J., Caldeira, R.L., Zhou, X.-N., 2018. Morphological and molecular characterization of invasive *Biomphalaria straminea* in southern China. Infect. Dis. Poverty 7, 120.

Hu, Q.-A., Zhang, Y., Guo, Y.-H., Lv, S., Xia, S., Liu, H.-X., Fang, Y., Liu, Q., Zhu, D., Zhang, Q.-M., Yang, C.-L., Lin, G.-Y., 2018. Small-scale spatial analysis of intermediate and definitive hosts of *Angiostrongylus cantonensis*. Infect. Dis. Poverty 7, 100.

Hung, N.M., Do, T.D., Anh, N.T.L., Van, P.T., Thanh, B.N., Van Ha, N., Van Hien, H., Le, X.C., 2015. Current status of fish-borne zoonotic trematode infections in Gia Vien district, Ninh Binh province, Vietnam. Parasit. Vectors 8, 21.

Jia, T.W., Wang, W., Sun, L.P., Lv, S., Yang, K., Zhang, N.M., Huang, X.B., Liu, J.B., Liu, H.C., Liu, R.H., Gawish, F.A., Habib, M.R., El-Emam, M.A., King, C.H., Zhou, X.N., 2019. Molluscicidal effectiveness of Luo-Wei, a novel plant-derived molluscicide, against Oncomelania hupensis, Biomphalaria alexandrina and Bulinus truncatus. Infect. Dis. Poverty 8 (1), 27. Erratum in: *Infect Dis Poverty* 2019, 8(1):42.

Jiang, B., Zhou, X.N., Zhang, H.B., Tao, Y., Huo, L.L., Liu, N., 2017. Slow-release praziquantel for dogs: presentation of a new formulation for echinococcosis control. Infect. Dis. Poverty 6 (1), 140.

Jiz, M., Wu, H.W., Meng, R., et al., 2008. Pilot-scale production and characterization of paramyosin, a vaccine candidate for schistosomiasis japonica. Infect Immun. 76, 3164–3169.

Khieu, V., Or, V., Tep, C., Odermatt, P., Tsuyuoka, R., Char, M.C., Brady, M.A., Sidwell, J., Yajima, A., Huy, R., Ramaiah, K.D., Muth, S., 2018. How elimination of lymphatic filariasis as a public health problem in the Kingdom of Cambodia was achieved. Infect. Dis. Poverty 7, 15.

Li, S.-Z., Qian, M.-B., Zhang, L.-J., Zhou, X.-N., 2007. Changing trends of neglected tropical diseases in China. The Lancet Infectious Diseases 17, 901.

Li, H.-M., Qian, M.-B., Yang, Y.-C., Jiang, Z.-H., Wei, K., Chen, J.-X., Chen, J.-H., Chen, Y.-D., Zhou, X.-N., 2018. Performance evaluation of existing immunoassays for *Clonorchis sinensis* infection in China. Parasit. Vectors 11, 35.

Liu, L., Yang, G.-J., Zhu, H.-R., Yang, K., Ai, L., 2014. Knowledge of, attitudes towards, and practice relating to schistosomiasis in two subtypes of a mountainous region of the People's Republic of China. Infect. Dis. Poverty 3, 16.

Miyamoto, K., Kirinoki, M., Matsuda, H., Hayashi, N., Chigusa, Y., Sinuon, M., Chuor, C.M., Kitikoone, V., 2014. Field survey focused on *Opisthorchis viverrini* infection in five provinces of Cambodia. Parasitol. Int. 63, 366–373.

Olveda, D.U., Olveda, R.M., McManus, D.P., Cai, P., Chau, T.N.P., Lam, A.K., Li, Y., Harn, D.A., Vinluan, M.L., Ross, A.G.P., 2014a. The chronic enteropathogenic disease schistosomiasis. Int. J. Infect. Dis. 28, 193–203.

Olveda, D.U., Olveda, R.M., Montes, C.J., Chy, D., Abellera III, J.M.B., Cuajunco, D., Lam, A.K., McManus, D.P., Li, Y., Ross, A.G.P., 2014b. Clinical management of advanced schistosomiasis: a case of portal vein thrombosis-induced splenomegaly requiring surgery. BMJ Case Rep. https://doi.org/10.1136/bcr-2014-203897.

Olveda, D.U., Olveda, R.M., Lam, A.K., Chau, T.N.P., Li, Y., Angelo Don Gisparil, I.I., Ross, A.G.P., 2014c. Utility of diagnostic imaging in the diagnosis and management of Schistosomiasis. Clin Microbial 3, 2. https://doi.org/10.4172/2327-5073.1000142.

Olveda, D.U., Li, Y., Olveda, R.M., Lam, A.K., McManus, D.P., Chau, T.N.P., Harn, D.A., Williams, G.M., Gray, D.J., Ross, A.G.P., 2014d. Bilharzia in the Philippines: past, present, and future. Int. J. Infect. Dis. 18, 52–56.

Olveda, D.U., Inobaya, M., Olveda, R.M., Vinluan, M.L., Ng, S.-K., Weerakoon, K., McManus, D.P., Ramm, G.A., Harn, D.A., Li, Y., Lam, A.K., Guevarra, J.R., Ross, A.G., 2017. Diagnosing schistosomiasis-induced liver morbidity: implications for global control. Int. J. Infect. Dis. 54, 138–144.

Pakharukova, M.Y., Vavilin, V.A., Sripa, B., Laha, T., Brindley, P.J., Mordvinov, V.A., 2015. Functional analysis of the unique cytochrome P450 of the liver fluke *Opisthorchis felineus*. PLoS Negl. Trop. Dis. 9, e0004258. https://doi.org/10.1371/journal.pntd.0004258.
Qian, M.-B., Zhou, X.-N., 2017. Global burden of cancers attributable to liver flukes. Lancet 5, e139.
Qian, M.-B., Zhou, X.-N., 2018. Walk together to combat echinococcosis. Lancet 18, 946.
Qian, M.-B., Chen, Y.-D., Fang, Y.-Y., Xu, L.-Q., Zhu, T.-J., Tan, T., Zhou, C.-H., Wang, G.-F., Jia, T.-W., Yang, G.-J., Zhou, X.-N., 2011. Disability Weight of Clonorchis sinensis infection: captured from community study and model simulation. PLoS Negl. Trop. Dis. 5 (12), e1377.
Qian, M.-B., Chen, Y.-D., Fang, Y.-Y., Tan, T., Zhu, T.-J., Zhou, C.-H., Wang, G.-F., Xu, L.-Q., Zhou, X.-N., 2013a. Epidemiological profile of *Clonorchis sinensis* infection in one community, Guangdong, People's Republic of China. Parasit. Vectors 6, 194.
Qian, M.-B., Chen, Y.-D., Yan, F., 2013b. Time to tackle clonorchiasis in China. Infect. Dis. Poverty 2, 4.
Qian, M.-B., Xia, S., Zhou, X.-N., 2015. Soil-transmitted helminths in China. Lancet 15, 1262–1263.
Ross, A.G.P., Olveda, R.M., Chy, D., Olveda, D.U., Li, Y., Harn, D.A., Gray, D.J., McManus, D.P., Tallo, V., Chau, T.N.P., 2015. Can mass drug administration lead to the sustainable control of schistosomiasis? J Infect Dis 211 (2), 283–289. https://doi.org/10.1093/infdis/jiu416.
Shi, F., Zhang, Y., Lin, J., Zuo, X., Shen, W., Cai, Y., Ye, P., Bickle, Q.D., Taylor, M.G., 2002. Field testing of *Schistosoma japonicum* DNA vaccines in cattle in China. Vaccine 20 (31 – 32), 3629–3631.
Sithithaworn, P., Andrews, R.H., Van De, N., Wongsaroj, T., Sinuon, M., Odermatt, P., Nawa, Y., Liang, S., Brindley, P.J., Sripa, B., 2012. The current status of opisthorchiasis and clonorchiasis in the Mekong basin. Parasitol. Int. 61, 10–16.
Sripa, B., Tangkawattana, S., Laha, T., Kaewkes, S., Mallory, F.F., Smith, J.F., Wilcox, B.A., 2015. Toward integrated opisthorchiasis control in Northeast Thailand: the Lawa project. Acta Trop. 141, 361–367.
Sripa, B., Deenonpoe, R., Brindley, P.J., 2017. Co-infections with liver fluke and *Helicobacter* species: a paradigm change in pathogenesis of opisthorchiasis and cholangiocarcinoma? Parasitol. Int. 66 (4), 383–389. https://doi.org/10.1016/j.parint.2016.11.016.
Tong, Q.-B., Chen, R., Zhang, Y., Yang, G.-J., Kumagai, T., Furushima-Shimogawara, R., Lou, D., Yang, K., Wen, L.-Y., Lu, S.-H., Ohta, N., Zhou, X.-N., 2015. A new surveillance and response tool: risk map of infected *Oncomelania hupensis* detected by loop-mediated isothermal amplification (LAMP) from pooled samples. Acta Trop. 141, 170–177.
Torgerson, P.R., Devleesschauwer, B., Praet, N., Speybroeck, N., Willingham, A.L., Kasuga, F., Rokni, M.B., Zhou, X.-N., Fèvre, E.M., Sripa, B., Gargouri, N., Fürst, T., Budke, C.M., Carabin, H., Kirk, M.D., Angulo, F.J., Havelaar, A., de Silva, N., 2015. World health organization estimates of the global and regional disease burden of 11 foodborne parasitic diseases, 2010: a data synthesis. PLoS Med. 12, e1001920. https://doi.org/10.1371/journal.pmed.1001920.
Wieringa, F.T., Dahl, M., Chamnan, C., Poirot, E., Kuong, K., Sophonneary, P., Sinuon, M., Greuffeille, V., Hong, R., Berger, J., Dijkhuizen, M.A., Laillou, A., 2016. The High Prevalence of Anemia in Cambodian children and women cannot be satisfactorily explained by nutritional deficiencies or hemoglobin disorders. Nutrients 8, 348. https://doi.org/10.3390/nu8060348.
Wu, H.W., Fu, Z.-Q., Lub, K., Pond-Tor, S., Meng, R., Hong, Y., Chu, K., Li, H., Jiz, M., Liu, J.-M., Hou, M., Park, S., Lin, J.-J., Kurtis, J.D., 2017. Vaccination with recombinant paramyosin in Montanide ISA206 protects against Schistosoma japonicum infection in water buffalo. Vaccine, Article in press.

Xu, J., Xu, J.-F., Li, S.-Z., Zhang, L.-J., Wang, Q., Zhu, H.-H., Zhou, X.-N., 2015. Integrated control programmes for schistosomiasis and other helminth infections in P.R. China. Acta Trop. 141, 332–341.
Yang, G.-J., Sun, L.-P., Hong, Q.-B., Zhu, H.-R., Yang, K., Gao, Q., Zhou, X.-N., 2012a. Optimizing molluscicide treatment strategies in different control stages of schistosomiasis in the People's Republic of China. Parasit. Vectors 5, 260.
Yang, J., Fu, Z., Feng, X., Shi, Y., Yuan, C., Liu, J., Hong, Y., Li, H., Lu, K., Lin, J., 2012b. Comparison of worm development and host immune responses in natural hosts of *Schistosoma japonicum*, yellow cattle and water. BMC Vet. Res. 8, 25.
Yang, G.-J., Utzinger, J., Zhou, X.-N., 2013a. Interplay between environment, agriculture and infectious diseases of poverty: case studies in China. Acta Trop. 141, 399–406. https://doi.org/10.1016/j.actatropica.2013.07.009.
Yang, K., Sun, L.-P., Liang, Y.-S., Wu, F., Li, W., Zhang, J.-F., Huang, Y.-X., Hang, D.-R., Liang, S., Bergquist, R., Zhou, X.-N., 2013b. Schistosoma japonicum risk in Jiangsu province, People's Republic of China: identification of a spatio-temporal risk pattern along the Yangtze River. Geospat. Health 8 (1), 133–142.
Yang, K., Zhou, X.-N., Jia, T.-W., Yang, G.-J., Wu, X.-H., Shi, X.-W., Li, H.-J., Steinmann, P., Utzinger, J., Bergquist, R., 2014. Eco-social determinants of Schistosoma japonicum infection supported by multi-level modelling in Eryuan County, People's Republic of China. Acta Trop. 141, 391–398. https://doi.org/10.1016/j.actatropica.2014.04.013.
Zhang, J.-F., Xu, J., Bergquist, R., Yu, L.-L., Yan, X.-L., Zhu, H.-Q., Wen, L.-Y., 2016. Development and application of diagnostics in the National Schistosomiasis Control Programme in the People's Republic of China. Adv. Parasitol. 92, 409–434. https://doi.org/10.1016/bs.apar.2016.02.008.
Zhou, X.-N., Lv, S., Yang, G.-J., Kristensen, T.K., Robert Bergquist, N., Utzinger, J., Malone, J.B., 2009. Meeting report: spatial epidemiology in zoonotic parasitic diseases: insights gained at the 1st international symposium on geospatial health in Lijiang, China, 2007. Parasit. Vectors 2, 10. https://doi.org/10.1186/1756-3305-2-10.
Zhu, Y., He, W., Liang, Y., Xu, M., Yu, C., Hua, W., Chao, G., 2002. Development of a rapid, simple dipstick dye immunoassay for schistosomiasis diagnosis. J. Immunol. Methods 266, 1–5.
Zhu, H.-R., Liu, L., Zhou, X.-N., Yang, G.-J., 2015. Ecological model to predict potential habitats of *Oncomelania hupensis*, the intermediate host of *Schistosoma japonicum* in the mountainous regions, China. PLoS Negl. Trop. Dis. 9, e0004028. https://doi.org/10.1371/journal.pntd.0004028.
Ziegler, A.D., Petney, T.N., Grundy-Warr, C., Andrews, R.H., Baird, I.G., Wasson, R.J., Sithithaworn, P., 2013. Dams and disease triggers on the lower Mekong river. PLoS Negl. Trop. Dis 7 (6), e2166. https://doi.org/10.1371/journal.pntd.0002166.

Further reading

Han, X.M., Cai, Q.G., Wang, W., Wang, H., Zhang, Q., Wang, Y.S., 2018. Childhood suffering: hyper endemic echinococcosis in Qinghai-Tibetan primary school students, China. Infect. Dis. Poverty 7 (1), 71.
Li, S.-Z., Qian, M.-B., Zhang, L.-J., Zhou, X.-N., 2017. Changing trends of neglected tropical diseases in China. Lancet 17, 901.
Li, B., Quzhen, G., Xue, C.Z., Han, S., Chen, W.Q., Yan, X.L., Li, Z.J., Quick, M.L., Huang, Y., Xiao, N., Wang, Y., Wang, L.Y., Zuoga, G., Bianba, G., Ma, B.C., Gasong, W.X.G., Niji, Z.C.J., Wu, W.P., Zhou, X.N., 2019. Epidemiological survey of echinococcosis in Tibet autonomous region of China. Infect. Dis. Poverty 8 (1), 29.

Liu, L., Guo, B., Li, W., Zhong, B., Yang, W., Li, S.C., Wang, Q., Zhao, X., Xu, K.J., Qin, S.C., Huang, Y., Yu, W.J., He, W., Liao, S., Wang, Q., 2018. Geographic distribution of echinococcosis in Tibetan region of Sichuan Province, China. Infect. Dis. Poverty 7 (1), 104.

Tambo, E., Ai, L., Zhou, X., Chen, J.-H., Hu, W., Bergquist, R., Guo, J.-G., Utzinger, J., Tanner, M., Zhou, X.-N., 2014. Surveillance-response systems: the key to elimination of tropical diseases. Infect. Dis. Poverty 3, 17.

Zhu, Y.-C., Socheat, D., Bounlu, K., Liang, Y.-S., Sinuon, M., Insisiengmay, S., He, W., Xu, M., Shi, W.-Z., Bergquist, R., 2005. Application of dipstick dye immunoassay (DDIA) kit for the diagnosis of schistosomiasis mekongi. Acta Trop. 96, 137–141.

CHAPTER FIVE

Multi-disciplinary integration of networking through the RNAS$^+$: Research on other target diseases

Lydia Leonardo[a,*], Robert Bergquist[b], Shi-Zhu Li[c,d,e,f,g], Shan Lv[c,d,e,f,g], Virak Khieu[h], Somphou Sayasone[i], Jing Xu[c,d,e,f,g], Remigio Olveda[j], Juerg Utzinger[k], Banchob Sripa[l], Fadjar Satrija[m], Sirikachorn Tangkawattana[l], Helena Ullyartha[n], Khin Thet Wai[o], Hung Nguyen[p], Xiao-Nong Zhou[c,d,e,f,g]

[a]Institute of Biology, College of Science, University of the Philippines Diliman and University of the East Ramon Magsaysay Graduate School, Quezon City, Philippines
[b]Geospatial Health, Ingerod, Brastad, Sweden
[c]National Institute of Parasitic Diseases, Chinese Center for Disease Control and Prevention, Shanghai, China
[d]Chinese Center for Tropical Diseases Research, Shanghai, China
[e]WHO Collaborating Centre for Tropical Diseases, Shanghai, China
[f]National Center for International Research on Tropical Diseases, Shanghai, China
[g]Key Laboratory of Parasite and Vector Biology, Ministry of Health, Shanghai, China
[h]National Helminth Control Program, National Center for Parasitology, Entomology and Malaria Control, Ministry of Health, Phnom Penh, Cambodia
[i]Lao Tropical and Public Health Institute, Vientianne, Lao People's Democratic Republic
[j]Asian Tropical Foundation, Filinvest Corporate City, Research Institute for Tropical Medicine Compound, Muntinlupa, Philippines
[k]Swiss Tropical and Public Health Institute, Basel, Switzerland
[l]Department of Pathology, Khon Kaen University, Khon Kaen, Thailand
[m]Bogor Agricultural University (IPB), JL. Agatis, Kampus IPB, Bogor, Indonesia
[n]Ministry of Health, South Jakarta, Indonesia
[o]Department of Medical Research, Ministry of Health & Sports, Yangon, Myanmar
[p]Department of Parasitology, Institute of Ecology and Biological Resources, Vietnam Academy of Science and Technology, Hanoi, Vietnam
*Corresponding author: e-mail address: lydialeonardo1152@gmail.com

Contents

1. Introduction 96
2. Neglected tropical diseases under the network 97
3. Food-borne trematodiases 98
4. Echinococcosis and cysticercosis 104
5. Lymphatic filariasis, soil-transmitted helminthiases and other helminthiases 105
References 108
Further reading 110

Advances in Parasitology, Volume 105
ISSN 0065-308X
https://doi.org/10.1016/bs.apar.2019.07.010

Abstract

In 2005, the network decided to increase its number of target diseases to include other helminthic zoonoses such as fascioliasis, clonorchiasis, opisthorchiasis, paragonimiasis and cysticercosis and in the process expanding membership to include South Korea, Vietnam, Thailand and Japan. NTDs were eventually included as awareness is heightened on these diseases affecting poor and developing countries. Researches on clonorchiasis and opisthorchiasis unravel the mechanism by which these diseases eventually predispose to cholangiocarcinoma. The liver cancer associated with these liver fluke infections necessitate the need to clarify the global burden of disease of these infections. The magnitude of these liver fluke diseases in endemic countries like China, Vietnam, Laos, Cambodia and Thailand is described. Success in elimination of lymphatic filariasis in PR China and Cambodia is highlighted to show how intensified multisectoral collaboration and strong political become strong ingredients in elimination of parasitic diseases like LF. New advances are presented that clarify species and strain differences in *Fasciola* spp., *Paragonimus* spp., *Taenia* spp. and *Echinococcocus* spp. Conventional diagnostic techniques are compared with new serologic techniques that are being developed. New control strategies such as the Lawa model are presented.

1. Introduction

When the network, at its fifth meeting held in Bali, Indonesia August 8–10, 2005, decided to include fascioliasis, clonorchiasis, cysticercosis, opisthorchiasis and paragonimiasis, besides schistosomiasis, it paved the way for adding Japan, South Korea, Thailand, and Vietnam and a change of name to the Regional Network on Asian Schistosomiasis and other Helminthic Zoonoses or RNAS^{+}. At its ninth meeting in Vientiane, Lao PDR October 19–20, 2009, the target diseases were further increased to include any NTD endemic in a member country. At this meeting, RNAS^{+} also drafted a programme to fit WPRO's Research Strategic Plan, identifying issues and operational research priorities, reassessing its role, defining strategies and future plans in contributing to the development of functional research on neglected tropical diseases (NTDs) in Asia. This chapter presents advances made with respect to target diseases, in particular those contributing to a better understanding of the epidemiology, pathogenesis, diagnosis, treatment and prevention and control of target diseases, mainly food-borne trematodiasis (FBTs), echinococcosis, cysticercosis, but also other NTDs.

2. Neglected tropical diseases under the network

Zhou et al. (2009) reported the results of the 1st International Symposium on Geospatial Health which was held in Lijiang, Yunnan province, People's Republic of China from 8 to 9 September 2007. The aim of the conference was to review progress made with the application of spatial techniques on zoonotic parasitic diseases, particularly in Southeast Asia. There were 71 presentations delivered on various parasitic diseases such as soil-transmitted and waterborne helminth infections and arthropod-borne diseases such as leishmaniasis, malaria and lymphatic filariasis. Various approaches in the study of these diseases were highlighted such as geographical information systems (GIS), global positioning systems (GPS) and remote sensing (RS), including spatial statistics, web-based GIS and map visualization of field investigations.

Tambo et al. (2014) presented the results of the "First Forum on Surveillance-Response System Leading to Tropical Diseases Elimination" which was held in Shanghai in June 2012 for the purpose of identifying and prioritizing strategic research on elimination of tropical diseases. Following a review of the current strategies and the NTD roadmap, identification and critical examination of the prevailing challenges and opportunities that include inter-sectoral collaboration and approaches for elimination of several infectious, tropical diseases, a priority research agenda was developed that involved a "One Health-One World" framework of global health. This research agenda included (i) the establishment of a platform for resource-sharing and effective surveillance-response systems for Asia Pacific and Africa with an initial focus on elimination of lymphatic filariasis, malaria and schistosomiasis; (ii) development of new strategies, tools and approaches, such as improved diagnostics and antimalarial therapies; and (iii) rigorous validation of surveillance-response systems; and (iv) designing pilot studies to transfer Chinese experiences of successful surveillance-response systems to endemic countries with limited resources.

Yang et al. (2015) made a review of emerging and re-emerging diseases like schistosomiasis, dengue, avian influenza, angiostrongyliasis and soil-transmitted helminthiasis that have affected China as a result of environmental and agricultural change. The association between poverty and infectious diseases is further influenced by environmental changes, agricultural practices and social status affecting emerging and re-emerging diseases such as schistosomiasis, dengue, avian influenza, and angiostrongyliasis. The group underscored research priorities and response strategies especially those involving mitigation and adaptation to eliminate re-emergence of these infectious diseases.

3. Food-borne trematodiases

Food-borne diseases (FBTs), transmitted through contaminated food, are important worldwide because of the significant mortality and morbidity especially in low and middle income countries where they contribute to high burdens of disease. A study of Torgerson et al. (2010) estimates the global and regional human disease burden of 10 helminth diseases and toxoplasmosis acquired by contaminated food. The results could pave the way to understanding the impact of FBTs globally and regionally. The study also indicates that the disease burden from most these parasites is highly focal but can lead to significant morbidity and mortality among vulnerable populations.

Human liver fluke infections caused by *Opisthorchis viverrini*, *O. felineus* and *C. sinensis* persist as significant public health problems in many countries world-wide especially in Asia. *C. sinensis* can be found in the southern part of PR China, South Korea and northern Vietnam, while *O. viverrini* is confined to the lower Mekong Basin, including Thailand, Lao PDR, Cambodia and central Vietnam. *O. felineus* is endemic in the former Soviet (USSR) and in Central–Eastern Europe. Recent estimates put a total of 700 million people at risk of clonorchiasis and opisthorchiasis. Qian et al. (2013c) compare clonorchiasis with hepatitis B which infects 23 million in China. Both diseases show higher prevalence among adult males compared to females and children. Both cause liver disease and impaired biliary conditions and produce similar symptoms such as fatigue, loss of appetite, fever, nausea, abdominal pain, jaundice and hepatomegaly. Both lead to liver cancer.

Qian et al. (2019) pointed out the importance of cooperation between PR China and Association of Southeast Asian Nations (ASEAN) in fight against human liver flukes. It is argued that $RNAS^+$ significantly provides important platform for further cooperation.

The first case of *C. sinensis* infection was found in 1874, which was completely documented in the Lancet in 1875. Thus, in the 140 years' anniversary of the discovery of the fluke, Qian et al. (2015) carried out a complete review on clonorchiasis in the Lancet. The seminar held for this purpose summarized the advance in clinical manifestations and complications, pathogenesis and carcinogenesis, epidemiology, environmental determinants and social-ecological systems, diagnosis, treatment and control of clonorchiasis. This disease is a common FBT in Southeast Asia including China, South Korea and Viet Nam where the estimates amount to 15 million infected people with populations at risk exceeding 600 million. However, the disease which is acquired by consumption of raw infected fish can also be found in countries where immigrants from endemic countries live. Chronic infections result in mild to serious sequelae leading to modification of the liver parenchyma with thickening and expansion of ducts including the gallbladder wall. However, this infection eventually develops into cholangiocarcinoma. Based on results of several studies on the association between *C. sinensis* infection and this type of cancer, this liver fluke was in 2009 considered as "carcinogenic to humans" (Group 1) by the International Agency for Research on Cancer (IARC). Still, clonorchiasis remains a NTD due to lack of paucity of information about the true disease burden, in particular the lack of a reliable disability-adjusted life year (DALY) score.

The study by Qian et al. (2013c) was the first attempt to calculate this showing that *C. sinensis* infection causes apparent disability. A positive correlation between disability and infection intensity was found and the overall score for the male is higher than that for the female. It is hoped that the disability determined in this study would pave the way for further studies facilitating a final estimation of disease burden to be used as basis for promoting health awareness and implementation of intervention. Qian and Zhou (2017) recently concluded that inadequate studies, incomplete data including the complex and chronic characteristics of cancers have not been helpful in determining an accurate estimate of the number of cholangiocarcinoma cases that can be attributed to liver flukes. Thus, it is important that more research be conducted in this field so as to raise awareness of the importance of these flukes in east Asia that will eventually lead to promotion of their control and elimination.

In PR China, where clonorchiasis is an important public health problem, comprehensive intervention strategies based on chemotherapy using praziquantel were implemented in the two endemic counties with the highest prevalence rates in 2006. The study of (Qian et al., 2013b) in one county in Guangdong showed differences in knowledge, behaviour and infection intensity among different populations necessitating the adoption of different intervention measurements for these different population groups. The group proposed that chemotherapy be prioritized among the adults especially adult males. Health education targeting children is seen to have a crucial role in the long term. Immigrants similarly should also be involved as well as restaurants that serve raw fish dish. Given the serious sequelae resulting from chronic infections with *C. sinensis*, early case management and treatment depend crucially on accurate and rapid diagnosis. Qian et al. (2013a) evaluated the diagnostic performance of Kato-Katz method and Formalin-ether concentration technique (FECT) in a clinical trial demonstrating that the Kato-Katz method is more sensitive in a setting of low infection intensity after drug treatment. However, the sensitivity of conventional stool examination techniques is inadequate and compliance has also decreased. Li et al. (2018) conducted a parallel and systematic evaluation of the performance of available immunodiagnostic kits detecting clonorchiasis in China. Their results showed good performance of three immunodiagnosis kits targeting IgG antibody in detecting chronic *C. sinensis* infection. But the kits detecting IgM antibody did not perform well.

Although praziquantel developed in later 1970s shows good efficacy against *C. sinensis* infection, new drugs are needed. Tribendimidine, a new drug against soil-transmitted helminths (STH) approved by the Chinese administration department in 2004, has been shown, both in vivo and in vitro efficacy against *C. sinensis*. Two clinical trials were conducted in PR China, one carried out by Qian et al. (2013a) in Guangxi in 2012, the other in Hunan province. Particularly, the side effect was less in tribendimidine group. In the former, the cure rate of a single dose of tribendimidine (400 mg) was a slightly inferior to praziquantel (25 mg/kg, t.i.d), but the egg reduction rates were comparable. On the other hand, the side effects were lower in tribendimidine group. The latter trial showed an efficacy of a single dose of tribendimidine (400 mg) comparable to praziquantel (75 mg/kg divided into four doses over 2 days), and the efficacy increased significantly by the second praziquantel treatment. The results of the two trials agreed with regard to the lower side effect of tribendimidine. In addition, Qian et al. (2019) demonstrated the effectiveness of school-based behavioural intervention against the practice of consuming raw freshwater fish. It was demonstrated that through comprehensive education, the knowledge on control of clonorchiasis increased and the practice of raw freshwater fish consumption decreased significantly.

Sithithaworn et al. (2012) describe the present status and control of *O. viverrini* and *C. sinensis* infections in the Mekong Basin countries. Presentations from the session "96 Years of Opisthorchiasis" during the International Congress of Liver Flukes (2018) provided up-to-date data on prevalence and distribution. It was concluded that high endemicity persists in all endemic countries of the lower Mekong Basin including high levels of cholangiocarcinoma incidence in spite of decades of treatment and control efforts. The review by Sithithaworn et al. (2012) noted that lowlands have significantly higher prevalence of *O. viverrini* compared with highlands. The higher prevalence was associated with wetlands, flooding patterns and human movement and settlement prevailing in the lowlands. The group recommended a more collaborative effort among all related government sectors.

Like *C. sinensis, O. viverrini* infection is classified by the International Agency for Research on Cancer as a Group 1 carcinogen: definitely carcinogenic in humans. Sripa et al. (2017) reviewed latest results that try to explain the role of liver fluke associated *Helicobacter pylori* in hepatobiliary disease and malignancy. Previous studies show cholangiocarcinoma cases with concurrent *H. pylori* infection to manifest higher portal inflammation and biliary cell proliferation as determined by PCNA immunohistochemistry. Further studies have shown the presence of *H. pylori* in the gut epithelium of *O. viverrini* leading to the conclusion that this liver fluke possibly serves as a reservoir of *H. pylori* within the biliary system. Sripa et al. (2017) have further brought up the possibility of co-infection with *O. viverrini* and *H. pylori* being at the core of the liver fluke infection associated cholangiocarcinoma.

Poor prognosis and limited efficacy of chemotherapy characterize this disease. Chng et al. (2016) report findings that show how the unique microbial communities found in the bile duct, parasitic infections and the tissue microenvironment can interact with each other to eventually lead to development of cancer. The group found that a specific bacterial family Bifidobacteriaceae dominated other bacterial families like Enterobacteriaceae and Enterococcaceae in tumours associated with *O. viverrini* infections which provides a mechanistic link to the parasite. Further functional analysis and comparison of cholangiocarcinoma microbiomes (for example, in tumours associated with *O. viverrini* and in tumours not associated with parasitic infection) showed higher possibility to produce bile acids and ammonia in tumours associated with *O. viverrini* thus providing the link between the changed microbiota to carcinogenesis.

Opisthorchiasis is endemic in Thailand and Lao PDR where it is considered an important public health problem throughout the Mekong Basin. Miyamoto et al. (2013) clarified the status of this liver fluke infection in Cambodia by documenting the extent and distribution of *O. viverrini* infection there. An extensive survey of 55 villages revealed the presence of this infection in four Cambodian provinces. This research group recommends careful planning in the field surveys because of the influence of complex environmental factors in the distribution of the disease. A nationwide baseline survey is further recommended to clarify the status of the disease in the country.

O. felineus is one of the three species belonging to the family Opisthorchiidae that causes liver disease. While *O. viverrini* and *C. sinensis* are classified as group 1 agents and a major risk factor for cholangiocarcinoma by the International Agency for Research on Cancer, while the potential of *O. felineus* to cause cancer is not that clear. *O. felineus* used to be endemic only within the territory of the Russian Federation, especially in Western Siberia, the Ukraine, Byelorussia, Kazakhstan and the Baltic countries but has recently been observed to be increasing in European regions, including Italy where reports of outbreaks of acute cases have been made lately. This fluke causes 1 in 10 cases of opisthorchiasis worldwide.

Pakharukova et al. (2015) conducted the first functional study of the cytochrome P450 (CYP) enzyme of flatworms using *O. felineus*, which causes biliary tract diseases in Russia, Kazakhstan and central Europe. Only one CYP450 enzyme was identified in *O. felineus*. This enzyme belongs to a group of proteins that are specifically involved in the synthesis of physiologically active compounds, in drug metabolism, and in biotransformation of xenobiotics. These researchers concluded that this could be a promising drug target but should be further investigated especially in understanding the physiology of this liver fluke.

Gouveia et al. (2017) support the inclusion of *O. felineus* in the Group 1 list of biological carcinogens. First, novel oxysterol-like metabolites, markedly similar to oxysterol-like molecules known from *O. viverrini,* both in egg and adult developmental stages of *O. felineus* by liquid chromatography-mass spectroscopy. These metabolites were also found in the bile, sera, and urine of liver fluke-infected hamsters. Second, portal area enlargement, inflammation with severe periductal fibrosis and changes in the epithelium of the biliary tract characterized as biliary intraepithelial neoplasia were validated by histological analysis of liver sections from hamsters infected with *O. felineus*. These biochemical and histopathological evidences seen in *O. felineus* infection in the rodent model suggest induction of precancerous lesions conducive to malignancy.

In spite of Thailand's protracted history of FBT control with corresponding nationwide reduction in prevalence of opisthorchiasis, the northeastern provinces in Thailand continue to harbour high prevalence of the infection. Sripa et al. (2015) reported the introduction of a new strategy using the EcoHealth/One Health approach in the Lawa Lake area in Khon Kaen Province where most of the endemic areas are found. The programme entitled the "Lawa model" uses anthelminth treatment, novel intensive health education methods both in the communities and in schools, ecosystem monitoring and active community participation. Results show significant decline to one-third of the 50% baseline in the infection rate in more than 10 villages surrounding the lake. Infection rate in the fish intermediate host decreased also considerably to less than 1% from a baseline of 70%. At present, the Lawa model has been recognized not only nationally but also internationally and being extended to neighbouring countries of the Mekong Basin.

Paragonimiasis (flukes encapsulated in the lungs) is not well understood from the point of view on disabilities caused and the DALY score fluctuates in different global burden of disease (GBD) estimates. Feng et al. (2018), in a systematic review of clinical paragonimiasis cases, recomputed the disability weight of human paragonimiasis and conclude that this DALY needs to be reconsidered in the light of the availability of morbidity data and species variation. However, determining the disease burden from paragonimiasis requires further modification with significant implications for public health prioritization in research, monitoring, and control. Chen et al. (2004) concluded that populations of *P. skrjabini* from five provinces of China are different strains of this species. *P. szechuanensis* is not a separate species but may be a geographical strain of *P. skrjabini* and *P. miyazaki* may be synonymous with *P. skrjabini*.

FBT infections due to *C. sinensis* constitute a major public health problem in Vietnam with transmission by consumption of raw fish or fish products. Hung et al. (2015) report that results from an extensive cross-sectional study reveal that there are FBT hotspots that remain in spite of the awareness of people on the risks of eating raw fish. These researchers recommend that any strategy to control FBT should stress the serious consequence of these infections and the critical need to stop the habit of eating raw fish.

Fascioliasis caused by either *Fasciola hepatica* or *F. gigantica* is the most common helminth infection in ruminants all over the world. This disease commonly causes death among cattle and goats. Human fascioliasis however is rarely reported, except in some countries. Chen et al. (2013) report that, while fascioliasis is common among livestock in PR China, human cases however are rarely reported. An outbreak of human fascioliasis was however reported in Yunnan Province in 2011. Symptoms observed among the cases were intermittent fever, epigastric tenderness, and hepatalgia. Blood tests showed eosinophilia and ultrasound revealed tunnel-like lesions in the liver. Administration of triclabendazole, the drug of choice for fascioliasis, significantly improved the patients' condition. Animal surveys yielded prevalence of 28.6% in cattle and 26.0% in goats. Molecular analysis confirmed co-existence of *F. hepatica* and *F. gigantica*. It was proposed that the herb *Houttuynia cordata* was most likely the source of infections. Chen et al. (2013) recommend distribution of triclabendazole for treatment of fascioliasis.

4. Echinococcosis and cysticercosis

Echinococcosis and cysticercosis are parasitic zoonoses of global concern. Although they do not cause high mortality, they result in significant impairment of human health and also agricultural production resulting in poor quality of life. There are key socioeconomic and environmental factors that influence transmission of both diseases that include poorly developed public health programmes, low hygiene and education standards, inefficient medical and veterinary services; climatic and environmental situations that perpetuate the zoonotic life-cycles. Several international meetings and workshops, held in PR China from 1998 to 2001, have led to an understanding of the seriousness of these diseases resulting in the development of a strategy to control echinococcosis and cysticercosis. Ito et al. (2003) report that this strategy involves an inclusive method that relies on a systematic analysis of the local settings especially concerning differences in the cycle, ecology and ethology with regard to the animal hosts, and behavioural characteristics of the population at risk. In addition, the use of newly developed tools, such as immunodiagnostics, molecular tools and imaging techniques and the convergence of traditional control measures (slaughter control, anti-parasitic treatment and control of the definitive hosts and health education) and more recent developments such as vaccination of the intermediate hosts.

Neurocysticercosis caused by *Taenia solium* metacestode or cysticercus larvae is one of the most common parasitic diseases in the central nervous system. Increased immigration rates and frequency of travel to endemic areas have resulted in the re-emergence of this disease in many communities. Symptoms depend on the size, number of cysticercus larvae and their location in the brain including the stage of infection. Chung et al. (2005) in the first seroepidemiological study of cysticercosis in the Nabo, Guangxi Zhuang Autonomous Region, report results that imply that cysticercosis is only relatively endemic in this area, with behavioural and environmental practices of the community responsible for the continued transmission of this parasitic infection. Chung et al. (2005) suggest that control and prevention of this disease should consider cultural traditions including human behaviour and promote the use of dedicated latrines.

Qian and Zhou (2018) report on the "Belt and Road Network for the Elimination and Control of Echinococcosis and Cysticercosis" that was set up in Chengdu, PR China in latter part of 2017. The primary objective of the network is to establish capacity for the research and development necessary to reach the control targets for echinococcosis, as well as those for cysticercosis by 2030. This will be based on the commitment, coordination, and cooperation of all endemic countries and the international community. The Chengdu Declaration to combat echinococcosis and cysticercosis was signed by experts representing 13 countries. The network invites participation of more countries in Europe and Asia to fight echinococcosis together.

Following the increased awareness from Chinese government on control of echinococcosis, more tools are developed to combat this zoonotic helminth. Yu et al. (2017, 2018) report the application of the technique of bait delivery with praziquantel using unmanned aerial vehicle for canine deworming, which could save manpower, time and overall cost in areas highly endemic for echinococcosis. Jiang et al. (2017) developed an in situ slow-release formulation of praziquantel by subcutaneous injection, which should be capable of resisting new *Echinococcus* infections for at least 6 months. Li et al. (2007) point out that echinococcosis has been put on high priority with the western endemic areas being the focus of substantial control activities.

In 2004, Jiang et al. reported the presence of potential antigenic proteins specific for alveolar echinococcosis or cystic echinococcosis from among different antigens shared by the two species of *Echinococcus*. Results could pave the way for further identifying specific antigens for immunodiagnosis. Now, Jiang et al. (2004a) have cloned, expressed and serologically evaluated the Em 18 antigen gene of *Echinococcus multilocularis* for diagnostic purpose. Their results are promising showing specificity of Re Em 18 antigens for alveolar echinococcosis with serum antibody level showing good correlation with the course of the disease at the early stage. Similar results were shown by evaluation of the ReEm 18-1 and ReEm18-2 antigens.

5. Lymphatic filariasis, soil-transmitted helminthiases and other helminthiases

Lymphatic filariasis (LF), one of the NTDs and a major public health problem in many tropical and sub-tropical countries, was targeted by the World Health Organization (WHO) for elimination as a public health problem by 2020. There are three species of nematode filarial worms

(*Wuchereria bancrofti, Brugia malayi*, and *B. timori*) that are transmitted by different species of mosquitoes. LF was confirmed to be endemic in Cambodia in 1956 when infected mosquitoes were found in Kratie province. An extensive study in 2001 further confirmed the endemicity of both *Brugia malayi* and *Wuchereria bancrofti*. A national task force to set up policies and work out strategies for controlling and eliminating NTDs was organized in 2015 with the goal of eliminating LF by 2015. Khieu et al. (2018) gave an account of the work done to eliminate LF as a public health problem in Cambodia. This involved successful MDAs, development of health center capacity for patient care, including the gains from socioeconomic progress and other measures against vector-borne diseases and NTDs. In 2016, WHO declared Cambodia as having achieved LF elimination as a public health problem. In China, LF was eliminated much earlier in 2006 after decades of sustained efforts focused on multisectoral collaboration involving various departments of the government, intensified control, prevention and elimination programme for LF and continued and massive cooperation from endemic populations (De-jian et al., 2013).

Qian et al. (2015) discuss the possibility of interrupting transmission of STH in China. Rapid economic development and intensified helminth control activities have reduced greatly the prevalence of STH in China from 536 million infected in 1988–1992 to 129 million in 2001–2004. National surveillance data also indicate continuing decline hence the shift to a higher goal of interruption transmission of STH in China which is expected not only to benefit China but the whole world as well. The group recommend the implementation of an expanded surveillance system for STH to provide real time data needed to assess transmission interruption process and make necessary adjustments. Tarafder et al. (2011), using Kato-Katz technique in an epidemiological study, show how mistakes in misclassification can affect the association between soil-transmitted helminth infection and schistosomiasis in humans. Using a statistical technique to compute for epidemiological measures of association after correcting for the inaccuracy of the test, results indicate a major difference between epidemiological measures of association before and after the correction of the inaccuracy of the test. Following correction of the error in the test, STH infection was shown to have an association with an increase in the risk of infection with schistosomiasis. The public health implications of this finding may be significant since this means that the effective control of one helminth can result in the decrease in the occurrence of another and therefore bring about a reduction in the overall burden of worm infections in affected regions.

Ezeamama et al. (2005) quantified the effect of polyparasite infections, including multiple concurrent low intensity infections on anaemia and found that low-intensity polyparasite infections were correlated with increased odds of anaemia. Often, the frequency of concurrent infection with multiple parasite species is higher than single-species infections. Results of the study indicate that concurrent low-intensity infections with more than one parasite species can eventually lead to clinically significant morbidity. Ezeamama et al. (2005) also estimate the synergistic effect caused by helminth species in their combined effects on anaemia. For example, concurrent infections of hookworm and either *S. japonicum* or *T. trichiura* were correlated with increased levels of anaemia than would be expected if the effects of these species had only independent effects on this. These findings indicate that an integrated anti-helminth treatment programmes synchronized with deworming for *S. japonicum* and STHs could result in a bigger effect than additive benefit for reducing anaemia in helminth-endemic regions.

McManus et al. (2014) report on the development and successful trial of a health education package to prevent STH infections among students of Han Chinese primary school in Hunan province, PR China. Results of the trial showed the direct effect of health education in improving knowledge and awareness, and in changing hygiene behaviour. Additionally, it could further improve the understanding of the public health outcomes of a multi-component integrated control programme especially where health education can result in prevention of re-infection while periodic drug treatment brings down prevalence and morbidity.

Qian and Zhou (2018) systematically evaluated the education products aiming at control and prevention of helminthiases in China. It is demonstrated that massive education products have been established for helminthiases in China. Most the products came from Centers for Disease Control and Prevention and Institutes of Parasitic Diseases at provincial and county levels. High number of products targeted schistosomiasis and echinococcosis, which also showed high quality, while those aiming other helminthiases were limited and inadequate.

Angiostrongyliasis is a food-borne nematode acquired by ingestion of molluscan intermediate host infected by the third stage larvae of *Angiostrongylus cantonensis*. Rodents are the regular definitive hosts with molluscs as intermediate hosts. Hu et al. (2018) investigated the infection status and spatial distribution of the hosts which can be used as basis for developing strategy for the prevention and control of angiostrongyliasis. The group report the existence of spatial correlation and spatial clusters in the distribution of infected *Pomacea canaliculata* snails and rats. The maximum radius of spatial cluster areas of infected rats also coincided with the rats' sphere of activity. A geographically weighted regression (GWR) model was found more advantageous than the ordinary least squares regression (OLS) model in the spatial analysis of hosts of *A. cantonensis*. The results point out that the risk of angiostrongyliasis is clearly present in Nanao Island, PR China and that large-scale monitoring should be undertaken without delay.

References

Chen, M.G., Chang, Z.S., Cui, A.L., Blair, D., Zhang, Y.N., Chen, S.H., Feng, Z., 2004. DNA sequences of *Paragonimus skrjabini* populations from five provinces in China. Chin. Med. J. (Engl) 117 (2), 219–224.

Chen, J.-X., Chen, M.-X., Ai, L., Xu, X.-N., Jiao, J.-M., Zhu, T.-J., Su, H.-Y., Zang, W., Luo, J.-J., Guo, Y.-H., Lv, S., Zhou, X.-N., 2013. An outbreak of human fascioliasis gigantica in Southwest China. PLoS One 8 (8), e71520. https://doi.org/10.1371/journal.pone.0071520.

Chng, K.R., Chan, S.H., Ng, A.H.Q., Li, C., Jusakul, A., Bertrand, D., Wilma, A., Pin Choo, S., Tan, D.M.Y., Lim, K.H., Soetinko, R., Ong, C.K., Duda, D.G., Dima, S., Popescu, I., Wongkham, C., Feng, Z., Yeoh, K.G., Teh, B.T., Yongvanit, P., Wongkham, S., Bhudhisawasdi, V., Khuntikeo, N., Tan, P., Pairojkul, C., Ngeow, J., Nagarajan, N., 2016. Tissue microbiome profiling identifies an enrichment of specific enteric bacteria in *Opisthorchis viverrini* associated cholangiocarcinoma. EBioMedicine 8, 195–202.

Chung, J.-Y., Eom, K.S., Yang, Y., Li, X., Feng, Z., Rim, H.-J., Cho, S.-Y., Kong, Y., 2005. A seroepidemiological survey of *Taenia solium* cysticercosis in Nabo, Guangxi Zhuang autonomous region, China. Korean J. Parasitol. 43 (4), 135–139.

De-jian, S., Xu-li, D., Ji-hui, D., 2013. The history of the elimination of lymphatic filariasis in China. Infect. Dis. Poverty 2, 30.

Ezeamama, A.E., Friedman, J.F., Olveda, R.M., Acosta, L.P., Kurtis, J.D., Mor, V., McGarvey, S.T., 2005. Functional significance of low-intensity polyparasite helminth infections in anemia. J. Infect. Dis. 192, 2160–2170.

Feng, Y., Fürst, T., Liu, L., Yang, G.-J., 2018. Estimation of disability weight for paragonimiasis: a systematic analysis. Infect. Dis. Poverty 7, 110.

Gouveia, M.J., Pakharukova, M.Y., Laha, T., Sripa, B., Maksimova, G.A., Rinaldi, G., Brindley, P.J., Mordvinov, V.A., Amaro, T., Santos, L.L., da Costa, J.M.C., Vale, N., 2017. Infection with *Opisthorchis felineus* induces intraepithelial neoplasia of the biliary tract in a rodent model. Carcinogenesis 38 (9), 929–937.

Hu, Q.-A., Zhang, Y., Guo, Y.-H., Lv, S., Xia, S., Liu, H.-X., Fang, Y., Liu, Q., Zhu, D., Zhang, Q.-M., Yang, C.-L., Lin, G.-Y., 2018. Small-scale spatial analysis of intermediate and definitive hosts of *Angiostrongylus cantonensis*. Infect. Dis. Poverty 7, 100.

Hung, N.M., Dung, D.T., Anh, N.T.L., Van, P.T., Thanh, B.N., Van Ha, N., Van Hien, H., Canh, L.X., 2015. Current status of fish-borne zoonotic trematode infections in Gia Vien district, Ninh Binh province,Vietnam. Parasit. Vectors 8, 21. https://doi.org/10.1186/s13071-015-0643-6.

Ito, A., Urbani, C., Jiamin, Q., Vuitton, D.A., Dongchuan, Q., Heath, D.D., Craig, P.S., Zheng, F., Schantz, P.M., 2003. Control of echinococcosis and cysticercosis: a public health challenge to international cooperation in China. Acta Trop. 86, 3.

Jiang, L., Feng, Z., Xue, H.C., Xu, X.N., Qiu, L.S., 2004a. Gene cloning, expression and serological evaluation of diagnostic antigen Em18 for alveolar echinococcosis. Zhongguo Ji Sheng Chong Xue Yu Ji Sheng Chong Bing Za Zhi 22 (4), 193–198.

Jiang, B., Zhou, X.N., Zhang, H.B., Tao, Y., Huo, L.L., Liu, N., 2017. Slow-release praziquantel for dogs: presentation of a new formulation for echinococcosis control. Infect. Dis. Poverty 6 (1), 140.

Khieu, V., Or, V., Tep, C., Odermatt, P., Tsuyuoka, R., Char, M.C., Brady, M.A., Sidwell, J., Yajima, A., Huy, R., Ramaiah, K.D., Muth, S., 2018. How elimination of lymphatic filariasis as a public health problem in the Kingdom of Cambodia was achieved. Infect. Dis. Poverty 7, 15.

Li, S.-Z., Qian, M.-B., Zhang, L.-J., Zhou, X.-N., 2007. Changing trends of neglected tropical diseases in China. Lancet 17, 901.

Li, H.-M., Qian, M.-B., Yang, Y.-C., Jiang, Z.-H., Wei, K., Chen, J.-X., Chen, J.-H., Chen, Y.-D., Zhou, X.-N., 2018. Performance evaluation of existing immunoassays for *Clonorchis sinensis* infection in China. Parasit. Vectors 11, 35. https://doi.org/10.1186/s13071-018-2612-3.

McManus, D.P., Bieri, F.A., Li, Y.-S., Williams, G.M., Yuan, L.-P., Henglin, Y., Du, Z.-W., Clements, A.C.A., Steinmann, P., Raso, G., Yap, P., Magalhães, R.J.S., Stewart, D., Ross, A.G., Halton, K., Zhou, X.-N., Olveda, R.M., Tallo, V., Gray, D.J., 2014. Health education and the control of intestinal worm infections in China: a new vision. Parasit. Vectors 7, 344.

Miyamoto, K., Kirinoki, M., Matsuda, H., Hayashi, N., Chigusa, Y., Sinuon, M., Chuor, C.M., Kitikoon, V., 2013. Field survey focused on *Opisthorchis viverrini* infection in five provinces of Cambodia. Parasitol. Int. 63, 366–373.

Pakharukova, M.Y., Vavilin, V.A., Sripa, B., Laha, T., Brindley, P.J., Mordvinov, V.A., 2015. Functional analysis of the unique cytochrome P450 of the liver fluke *Opisthorchis felineus*. PLoS Negl. Trop. Dis. 9 (12), e0004258. https://doi.org/10.1371/journal.pntd.0004258.

Qian, M.-B., Zhou, X.-N., 2017. Global burden of cancers attributable to liver flukes. Lancet 5, PE139.

Qian, M.-B., Zhou, X.-N., 2018. Walk together to combat echinococcosis. Lancet Infect. Dis. 18 (9), 946.

Qian, M.-B., Chen, Y.-D., Yan, F., 2013a. Time to tackle clonorchiasis in China. Infect. Dis. Poverty 2, 4.

Qian, M.-B., Chen, Y.-D., Fang, Y.-Y., Tan, T., Zhu, T.-J., Zhou, C.-H., Wang, G.-F., Xu, L.-Q., Zhou, X.-N., 2013b. Epidemiological profile of *Clonorchis sinensis* infection in one community, Guangdong, People's Republic of China. Parasit. Vectors 6, 194.

Qian, M.-B., Chen, Y.-D., Fang, Y.-Y., Xu, L.-Q., Zhu, T.-J., Tan, T., Zhou, C.-H., Wang, G.-F., Jia, T.-W., Yang, G.-J., Zhou, X.-N., 2013c. Disability weight of *Clonorchis sinensis* infection: captured from community study and model simulation. Parasit. Vectors 6, 194.

Qian, M.-B., Xia, S., Zhou, X.-N., 2015. Soil-transmitted helminths in China. Lancet 15, 1262–1263.

Qian, M.B., Zhou, C.H., Zhu, H.H., Zhu, T.J., Huang, J.L., Chen, Y.D., Zhou, X.N., 2019. Assessment of health education products aimed at controlling and preventing helminthiases in China. Infect. Dis. Poverty 8 (1), 22.

Sithithaworn, P., Andrews, R.H., Van De, N., Wongsaroj, T., Sinuon, M., Odermatt, P., Nawa, Y., Liang, S., Brindley, P.J., Sripa, B., 2012. The current status of opisthorchiasis and clonorchiasis in the Mekong Basin. Parasitol. Int. 61, 10–16.

Sripa, B., Tangkawattana, S., Laha, T., Kaewkes, S., Mallory, F.F., Smith, J.F., Wilcox, B.A., 2015. Toward integrated opisthorchiasis control in Northeast Thailand: the Lawa Project. Acta Trop 141, 361–367.

Sripa, B., Deenonpoe, R., Brindley, P.J., 2017. Co-infections with liver fluke and Helicobacter species: a paradigm change in pathogenesis of opisthorchiasis and cholangiocarcinoma? Parasitol. Int. 66 (4), 383–389.
Tambo, E., Ai, L., Zhou, X., Chen, J.-H., Hu, W., Bergquist, R., Guo, J.-G., Utzinger, J., Tanner, M., Zhou, X.-N., 2014. Surveillance-response systems: the key to elimination of tropical diseases. Infect. Dis. Poverty 3, 17.
Tarafder, M.R., Carabin, H., McGarvey, S.T., Joseph, L., Balolong Jr., E., Olveda, R., 2011. Assessing the impact of misclassification error on an epidemiological association between two helminthic infections. PLoS Negl. Trop. Dis. 5 (3), e995. https://doi.org/10.1371/journal.pntd.0000995.
Torgerson, P.R., Devleesschauwer, B., Praet, N., Speybroeck, N., Willingham, A.L., Kasuga, F., Rokni, M.B., Zhou, X.-N., Fèvre, E.M., Sripa, B., Gargouri, N., Fürst, T., Budke, C.M., Carabin, H., Kirk, M.D., Angulo, F.J., Havelaar, A., de Silva, N., 2010. World Health Organization estimates of the global and regional disease burden of foodborne parasitic diseases, 2010: a data synthesis. PLoS Med. 12 (12), e1001920. https://doi.org/10.1371/journal.pmed.1001920.
Yang, G.-J., Utzinger, J., Zhou, X.-N., 2015. Interplay between environment, agriculture and infectious diseases of poverty: case studies in China. Acta Trop. 141 (Pt. B), 399–406.
Yu, Q., Xiao, N., Yang, S.J., Han, S., 2017. Deworming of stray dogs and wild canines with praziquantel-laced baits delivered by an unmanned aerial vehicle in areas highly endemic for echinococcosis in China. Infect. Dis. Poverty 6 (1), 117.
Yu, Q., Liu, H., Xiao, N., 2018. Unmanned aerial vehicles: potential tools for use in zoonosis control. Infect. Dis. Poverty 7 (1), 49.
Zhou, X.-N., Lv, S., Yang, G.-J., Kristensen, T.K., Robert Bergquist, N., Utzinger, J., Malone, J.B., 2009. Meeting report spatial epidemiology in zoonotic parasitic diseases: insights gained at the 1st international symposium on geospatial health in Lijiang, China. Parasit. Vectors 2, 10.

Further reading

Eom, K.S., Jeon, H.-K., Kong, Y., Hwang, U.W., et al., 2002. Identification of *Taenia asiatica* in China: molecular, morphological and epidemiological analysis of a Luzhai isolate. J. Parasitol. 88 (4), 758–764.
Ezeamama, A.E., McGarvey, S.T., Acosta, L.P., Zierler, S., Manalo, D.L., Wu, H.-W., Kurtis, J.D., Mor, V., Olveda, R.M., Friedman, J.F., 2008. The synergistic effect of concomitant schistosomiasis, hookworm, and *Trichuris* infections on children's anemia burden. PLoS Negl. Trop. Dis. 2 (6), e245. https://doi.org/10.1371/journal.pntd.0000245.
Jiang, L., Xue, H.C., Qiu, L.S., Feng, Z., 2004b. Western blotting analysis of specific antigens from different components of Echinoccocus metacestodes. Zhongguo Ji Sheng Chong Xue Yu Ji Sheng Chong Bing Za Zhi 22 (1), 11–15.
Sripa, B., Tangkawattana, S., Laha, T., Kaewkes, S., Mallory, F.F., Smith, J.F., Wilcox, B.A., 2014. Toward integrated opisthorchiasis control in Northeast Thailand: the Lawa project. Acta Trop. 141, 361–367.

CHAPTER SIX

From inspiration to translation: Closing the gap between research and control of helminth zoonoses in Southeast Asia

Robert Bergquist[a,*], Lydia Leonardo[b,c], Xiao-Nong Zhou[d,e,f,g,h]

[a]Geospatial Health, Ingerod, Brastad, Sweden
[b]Institute of Biology, College of Science, University of the Philippines Diliman, Quezon City, Philippines
[c]University of the East Ramon Magsaysay Graduate School, Quezon City, Philippines
[d]National Institute of Parasitic Diseases, Chinese Center for Disease Control and Prevention, Shanghai, China
[e]Chinese Center for Tropical Diseases Research, Shanghai, China
[f]WHO Collaborating Centre for Tropical Diseases, Shanghai, China
[g]National Center for International Research on Tropical Diseases, Shanghai, China
[h]Key Laboratory of Parasite and Vector Biology, Ministry of Health, China; Shanghai, China
*Corresponding author: e-mail address: robert.bergquist@outlook.com

Contents

1. Introduction 112
2. Research activities and raison d'être 114
3. International research funding 117
4. What is still missing? 118
5. Lessons learnt and the way forward 119

References 121

Abstract

Poverty magnifies limitations resulting from traditional biases and environmental risks in endemic areas. Any approach towards disease control needs to recognise that socially embedded vulnerabilities can be as powerful as externally imposed infections. Important for RNAS was networking across borders, not just on schistosomiasis but on the whole spectrum of endemic helminthiases, and this bore fruit in the form of the expansion of RNAS into the 'Regional Network on Asian Schistosomiasis and other Helminth Zoonoses (RNAS$^+$)', which focuses on technical standardization, supporting the growth of research capacity and the further development of networking. Administration is lean and largely virtual with the focus on connecting members via the Internet, providing databases and administrative back-up. The strategy emphasizes ways and means to alleviate the spectre of disease and poverty from the endemic areas through boosting research on target diseases and supporting collaboration between basic and operational research on the one hand and control/elimination activities on the other. RNAS$^+$ also benefits from continuing input from outside research institutions in areas outside Southeast Asia. This paper is aiming to identify the priority actions to close the gap between researcher and policy makers.

Advances in Parasitology, Volume 105
ISSN 0065-308X
https://doi.org/10.1016/bs.apar.2019.07.011

1. Introduction

Helminth infections constitute a considerable public health burden covering such diverse diseases as dracunculiasis echinococcosis, food-borne trematodes (FBTs), lymphatic filariasis (LF), onchocerciasis, soil-transmitted helminths (SHTs), schistosomiasis as well as *Strongyloides* and *Taenia* infections including cysticercosis. Trematodes and nematodes tend to be the most investigated parasitic worms, while work on cestodes is trailing. Thanks to the growing awareness of public health issues, Ministries of Health are gauging the economic impact of these diseases and considering political and financial commitments directed against the neglected tropical diseases (NTDs). Poverty magnifies limitations of any approach towards disease control and, like all tropical, poverty-stricken areas, Southeast Asia's panorama of parasitic diseases, have a tendency to emerge/re-emerge when control activities are not sustained. Only access to up-to-date data and support systems capable of locating high-risk areas can block the vicious circle of endemic presence of NTDs and poor people unable to work and provide for themselves and their families due to disease.

Thanks to the Internet and television, the world of today is fully aware of public health needs in low- and middle-income countries in the tropical part of the world. Governments, non-government organizations (NGOs) and donor foundations are all trying to improve the situation. For example, the World Health Organization (WHO) has developed a 'roadmap' for the elimination or strongly reducing the prevalence of the major endemic diseases within the current decade (WHO, 2012), a proposal endorsed by the World Health Assembly (WHA) resulting in the largest public health initiative in history. In London, UK, the same year, senior government officials in the industrial world together with their counterparts in the endemic countries, research institutions, universities, major donor organization and leading pharmaceutical industry corporations issued the *London Declaration* on the Neglected Tropical Diseases (https://unitingtocombatntds.org/london-declaration-neglected-tropical-diseases/). This joint commitment issued aims to: eradicate or prevent transmission of dracunculiasis (Guinea worm disease); eliminate LF, leprosy, African trypanosomiasis (sleeping sickness) and trachoma; and control American trypanosomiasis (Chagas), river blindness (onchocerciasis), schistosomiasis, STHs and visceral leishmaniasis. Inspired by these initiatives, universal health coverage has become a central component of the United Nations' 17 Sustainable Development

Goals (SDGs) for the period 2015–2030 (United Nations, 2015), which aims to bring today's 'medical toolbox' to bear on the NTDs and lift the burden of disease from all in countries currently lacking full access to health services.

Less than 7 years later, it is already clear that the situation has improved in a general way, making a more detailed view worthwhile. The treetops need to know what is going on at the grassroots level and this is where networking comes in. Stimulation of multi-disciplinary approaches for the control of endemic, helminth diseases in Southeast Asia by long-term input from the UNICEF/UNDP/World Bank/WHO Special Programme for Research and Training in Tropical Diseases (TDR) through the creation of the 'Regional Network on Asian Schistosomiasis (RNAS)' in the year 2000 was pivotal. This was not only a first attempt to improve interchange between national research institutes and research groups in the region, but also a way to promote collaboration between individual researchers and their counterparts working for national control programmes of various kinds. RNAS worked closely with the WHO Western Pacific Regional Office (WPRO) and benefitted also from ongoing parallel projects funded by the Rockefeller Foundation, the United States' (U.S.) National Institutes of Health (NIH) and the World Bank, while expanding its support base with dedicated grants from the Canadian International Development Research Centre (IDRC). Basic and operational research took off followed by investigation of new control strategies. Important for the activities encouraged by these initiatives was networking across borders, not just on schistosomiasis but on the whole spectrum of endemic helminthiases, and this bore fruit in the form of the expansion of RNAS into the 'Regional Network on Asian Schistosomiasis and other Helminth Zoonoses (RNAS^{+})'.

Activities started with a collaboration on schistosomiasis japonica between scientists in the People's Republic of China (PR China) and the Philippines, but as soon as the new network had been formed, it rapidly added Cambodia, Indonesia, the Lao People's Democratic Republic (Lao PDR) and Japan that were not much later joined by the Republic of Korea, Vietnam and Thailand and finally Myanmar. Meanwhile, clonorchiasis, cysticercosis, fascioliasis, opisthorchiasis, paragonimiasis and schistosomiasis mekongi were added to the roster. The network vision is to become the recognized platform for evidence-based information and communication bridging the gap between research scientists and control authorities for the prevention of NTDs in Southeast Asia. To that end, RNAS^{+} focuses on technical standardization, supporting the growth of research capacity and the development of networking. Administration is lean and largely virtual with the focus on connecting members via the Internet, providing databases and administrative back-up. The strategy emphasizes ways and means to alleviate the spectre of disease and poverty from the endemic areas through boosting research on its target diseases and supporting collaboration between basic and operational research on the one hand and control/elimination activities on the other. RNAS$^+$ also benefits from continuing input from outside research institutions in Australia, Denmark, Switzerland, the United Kingdom and United States.

2. Research activities and raison d'être

RNAS$^+$ has provided critical research with regard to several parasitic diseases common in the Southeast Asian region. Network members are involved in various fields disseminating information to the whole group as it is gained. Traditional epidemiological approaches are utilized as well as advanced, spatial statistics linked to the use of geographical information systems (GIS) and satellite-generated data (remote sensing). The basic line of investigations, such as operational research and implementation of evidence-based policies along with dedicated work on key technologies, such as advanced diagnostics, modelling and development of vaccines and new drugs continue to be key research objectives. Most of the tools needed for the different research activities are regularly taught at 1–2 day RNAS$^+$ training courses following the annual meetings and the new skills later applied in field and laboratory in collaboration with experienced scientists. Sometimes, separate, longer training activities have been held outside the region. For example, with respect to schistosomiasis in animals, a workshop on diagnostic tests was held in September 2003 at the Danish Bilharziasis Laboratory (DBL) in Copenhagen, Denmark. It had a wider participation than just from Southeast Asia but was attended by 16 participants connected with RNAS$^+$ from countries including Cambodia, PR China, Indonesia, Lao PDR and the Philippines. The purpose of the workshop was to demonstrate, compare and reach consensus about diagnostic tests to be used for surveys, control and surveillance on animal schistosomiasis in Asia (Olveda et al., 2010; Zhou et al., 2008).

The success achieved is based on an overall aim to strengthen collaboration between scientists and the authorities responsible for disease control in the endemic countries. The RNAS$^+$ framework, website, databases, publications and its annual meetings have helped building local technical standards and instituting mechanisms for information-sharing with emphasis on platform design and technical standardization fostering strengthened research capacity (Bergquist and Whittaker, 2012). RNAS$^+$'s administrative body is largely virtual connecting members via the Internet, providing background information (databases when available) and general back-up. The underlying philosophy is that the overall goal should benefit from the creation of interconnected disease-specific groups capable of operating as nodes accessible at the RNAS$^+$ website (http://www.rnas.org.cn). Brief introductions to commonly used approaches, such as GIS, modelling and diagnostics follow below.

The strength of GIS in the area of vector-borne diseases lies in the environmental vector requirements that limit these infections to highly specific ecological niches (Malone et al., 2016), and hidden relationships and patterns may be revealed by using location as the key index (Rinaldi et al., 2011). GIS generally uses data downloaded from satellites collecting environmental data on a continuous basis (Malone et al., 2019). This type of remote sensing can be utilized for the development of predictive models showing the association between environmental conditions and parasite prevalence. In addition, Google Earth and its web-based pendant Google Maps are conducive to combination of results from literature and field findings (Stensgaard et al., 2009; Twardzik et al., 2018). The concept of time geography, long ago advanced by Hägerstrand (1970), has now produced the space-time cube (STC), where the base represents a 2-D geographical map with the vertical axis treated as time instead of altitude. The revived interest in Hägerstrand's innovative idea eventually led to an ESRI application (https://support.esri.com/en/technical-article/000017460) where the visualized fusion of space and time facilitate understanding of the spread of diseases.

Mathematical modelling can help predicting the potential impact of a specific control intervention (Williams et al., 2019) and represents a way to understand reality by simplification. Although all models are by definition wrong, some capture essential features of reality more closely than others, which means that the data are better fitting. Depending on the question studied, a model should only be as complex as needed, an approach referred to as the principle of parsimony or Occam's razor after the British mediaeval thinker. However, the ecological dynamics of infections have a wide range of interconnected spatial scales, some are directly transmitted within a single species, whereas others circulate among multiple hosts. Even if this creates a situation where the mathematics become complex, modelling still offer valuable tools to understand the epidemiological patterns needed for deciding which strategy to implement (Heesterbeek et al., 2015).

$RNAS^+$ has a strong interest in diagnostic approaches for all its target diseases, but most work has been carried out on schistosomiasis. The daily variations in host egg excretion is particularly pronounced in *Schistosoma japonicum* infections (Yu et al., 1998) and can therefore result in falsely negative tests in areas characterized by low-intensity infection. The solution lies in modifying the methodology according to the diagnostic need (Bergquist et al., 2009), which means that a shift to a more sensitive and specific test is needed when the priority moves from traditional individual diagnosis and monitoring to surveillance and response in a well-controlled landscape. Today, disease and infection are diagnosed through the expression of biomarkers (http://www.biomarkersconsortium.org/). However, this concept varies from the vague, e.g. increased body temperature, to the specific, such as the demonstration of a schistosome egg. Both are biological markers, but NTD epidemiology deals with more narrow subsets, such as what is discovered by microscopy, immunological techniques, genomics or technologies that visualize pathology, e.g., ultrasonography.

The thick stool smear technique, originally described by Kato and Miura (1954) and later standardized by the introduction of a 41.7 mg template by Katz et al. (1972), is a standardized approach to helminth egg detection, but the miracidium hatching test for schistosomiasis diagnosis is widely used in PR China (Qiu and Xue, 1990). The sensitivity of the hatching technique is slightly better than the Kato-Katz technique, probably due to large volumes of faeces, but a combination of stool examination and hatching produces even better results (Zhu et al., 2014). The development of the dipstick dye immunoassay (DDIA) kit for schistosomiasis japonicum diagnosis (Zhu et al., 2002) and its subsequent successful application for community diagnosis of schistosomiasis mekongi in Cambodia and Lao PDR (Zhu et al., 2005) on the one hand, and the standardization of ultrasound findings in Asian schistosomiasis (Li et al., 2004) on the other, were promoted by $RNAS^+$ using funds from TDR.

There has also been progress involving highly sensitive diagnostic techniques, e.g., by using the loop-mediated isothermal amplification (LAMP) for surveying snails for schistosome infection (Qin et al., 2018) and application of the up-converting phosphor lateral flow (UCP-LF) technology for detection of *S. japonicum* and *S. mekongi* infection through the presence of circulating antigens (van Dam et al., 2015) as well as various variants of the polymerase chain reaction (PCR) (Cai et al., 2019; Weerakoon et al., 2018).

Vaccine development in Southeast Asia is quite different from the mainstream as it targets the reservoir hosts, such cattle and water buffaloes, which are the main culprits in sustaining the *S. japonicum* life cycle. For this reason, vaccination is a valid means to reduce the excretion of egg from domestic animals. A DNA-based vaccine (SjCTPI) has shown encouraging efficacy against *S. japonicum* in Chinese water buffaloes (Williams et al., 2019). This trial confirms that human praziquantel treatment is an effective intervention at the population level, while mollusciciding has an indirect ~50% efficacy in reducing human infection rates. A transmission blocking vaccine targeting bovines, such as the SjTPI for the prevention of *S. japonicum* with the required protective efficacy, would be invaluable in tandem with these and other preventive measures.

Studies on drugs against liver flukes and intestinal nematodes have shown the diamidine derivative tribendimidine, developed in the late 1980s by the National Institute of Parasitic Diseases (NIPD), to be a good candidate (Ren et al., 1987). Although the drug is ineffective with regard to *S. japonicum,* a collaboration was entered between NIPD and the Swiss Tropical and Public Health Institute (*Swiss TPH*) to screen it further. The drug was found to have a good effect against various helminths of the FBT group but schistosomes and *F. hepatica* were not affected (Keiser et al., 2007; Panic et al., 2014). The work continued within the $RNAS^+$ framework and tribendimidine is currently in advanced clinical trials against *Opisthorchis viverrini* (Sayasone et al., 2018).

3. International research funding

Core funding from WHO and TDR has helped to keep $RNAS^+$ supporting its annual meetings, but it was already clear from the beginning that it would in the longer term need outside funding from other sources as well. To that end several research proposals were developed. The interest from IDRC in Canada in one of these project resulted in a major grant and $RNAS^+$ was pleased to be awarded, a 3-year (2011–2014) multi-country, multi-institution project on ecological intervention approaches to interfere with transmission schistosomiasis and other zoonotic helminths. The general objective of this project was to develop innovative strategies for the sustainable control of target emerging infectious diseases through socio-ecosystem based interventions. The research was shared between by research institutions in Cambodia, Lao PDR, the Philippines, PR China; Thailand and Vietnam.

The main helminths identified as particular problems in the region were found to be STHs, schistosomiasis and the FBTs, but also cysticercosis, echinococcosis and LF are important in large areas. Three cluster zones corresponding to specific helminth groupings were identified and it was confirmed that livestock has the leading role with regard to transmission. Higher re-infection was observed both in humans and livestock, and the lack of multi-sectoral cooperation was noted. Lessons learnt from this project included the understanding that ecosystems govern helminth transmission overall and to move forward a classification system and identification of the hotspots are needed. Children, women and minorities were found to be the most vulnerable, but the importance of the information education and communication (IEC) component was difficult to measure. The lack of professional teams with trans-disciplinary and ecohealth knowledge was also noted. A follow-up IDRC-supported project involving Cambodia, Lao PDR, PR China and Thailand, dealt with the development of country-specific transformation frameworks to advance the elimination of schistosomiasis and effective control of schistosomiasis and liver fluke infections in the Greater Mekong sub region but final results are not yet available.

In addition, three specific projects were supported by TDR: (1) community diagnosis of schistosomiasis mekongi (Zhu et al., 2002); (2) standardization of ultrasonography in Asian schistosomiasis (Li et al., 2004); and development of survey tools for animal schistosomiasis (Olveda et al., 2010).

4. What is still missing?

Reliable, long-term information on mortality and life expectancy has not been much utilized by RNAS$^+$ members, but should be a good guiding principle when attempting to gauge the impact of the endemic diseases in the region. For purposes such as understanding public health trends, health metrics aims to find a single measure that summarizes the impact of both mortality and morbidity on health, e.g., finding a number between 0 (death) and 1 (optimal health) presents a complex methodological challenge. Available publications on this issue that appear under the measurement rubrics of health-adjusted life years provide helpful information, e.g., health-adjusted life expectancy (HALE), quality-adjusted life years (QALYs), years of healthy life (YHLs) and disability-adjusted life years (DALYs) (Field and Gold, 1998; Neiger et al., 2012; Murray et al., 2012).

There needs to be enhanced laboratory ability in areas with significant NTD prevalence to provide technical and scientific support for the diagnosis, surveillance, monitoring and evaluation of national NTD programmes (WHO, 2012). Diagnostic laboratory networks are informal and not well publicized making it difficult to share expertise and provide supervision and quality assurance as well as standardization. Such work has started in connection with $RNAS^+$ but is still not strong. Indeed, a very recent study commissioned by WHO found that although more than 90% of laboratories investigated had adequate technical skills to function as an NTD reference laboratory, almost all of them lacked systems for external verification (Dean et al., 2018). The WHO Strategic and Technical Advisory Group (STAG) for the NTDs therefore prioritizes strengthening laboratories and the establishment of a laboratory network capable of providing quality assurance. $RNAS^+$ could play an important role here by establishing rules for diagnostic assays and how they should be used and issue guidelines for reference laboratories.

Decisions regarding interventions require diagnostics to provide data on prevalence and intensity of helminth diseases. Importantly, diagnostic approaches need also detect signs indicating drug resistance. As referred to in previous chapters in this book, many different assays are applied in the region but, with exception of the Kato-Katz stool examination (Katz et al., 1972) for schistosomiasis stool examination, they are not well standardized (Dean et al., 2018), which would be helpful in comparing data from different areas and countries. Although laboratory services are decisive with respect to choice of intervention mode for control and surveillance, the technical staff in most low-resource settings are insufficiently trained (Nkengasong et al., 2010). Preventive chemotherapy through mass drug administration (MDA) not only relies on laboratory data for estimating initial prevalence, but this approach also requires knowledge of intervention effectiveness and documentation of progress. There has been progress with regard to schistosomiasis and also other NTDs. LF has been eliminated in Cambodia (Khieu et al., 2018) and PR China (De-Jian et al., 2013), while malaria is substantially reduced and close to elimination in China (Yin et al., 2013). Still, an accelerated scale-up of existing activities in this area is critical if the stated NTD Roadmap targets for 2020 are to be reached.

5. Lessons learnt and the way forward

In spite of the impressive success of reducing the number of schistosomiasis cases in PR China with more than 95% since the peak human prevalence in the mid-1950s with between 10.5 and 11.8 million (high-intensity) cases (Chen and Feng, 1999; Mao and Shao, 1982). A strong impetus had been added by the 1992–2001 World Bank Loan Project (WBLP) which particularly emphasized praziquantel-based morbidity control (Chen, 2005; Zhang et al., 2012). Although the progress momentarily stalled in the first years of the new millennium, further improvement ensued when snail control, that had been overshadowed by the strong focus on chemotherapy during the WBLP years, was again promoted (Utzinger et al., 2005). RNAS$^+$ was seen as the vehicle to translate the Chinese progress on schistosomiasis elimination into the Philippines, but it was soon realized that the situation in this country is radically different from that in PR China, partly because transmission is not seasonal as in PR China and partly because of the topography: large plains in PR China in contrast to the many islands that are often hilly and covered with wild, tropical vegetation in the Philippines. In addition, the integrated multidisciplinary campaigns used in PR China could not be duplicated in the Philippines because of limited financial resources (Olveda and Grey, 2019). In a global perspective, this is not so unlike the problem with schistosomiasis mansoni in southern and northern Brazil on the one hand, and the Mediterranean countries and sub-Saharan Africa on the other.

The collaboration between Chinese and Filipino researchers that started the network could not immediately breach these seemingly insurmountable differences between their countries, but discussions paved the way for an understanding that elimination cannot just be a question of praziquantel production and distribution. Apart from chemotherapy, a working control strategy must be based on a sustained political commitment to improve the situation (Chen et al., 2018; Maegraith, 1958), it should also be adapted to local eco-epidemiological settings and strangly hinge on a strong emphasis on snail control (Chen and Feng, 1999). Importantly, the WBLP was different from previous World Bank interventions in that a small part (3%) of the financial support was earmarked for research support (Utzinger et al., 2005). This component would eventually turn out to lead to outcomes that could be directly plugged into the ongoing schistosomiasis control activities. Therefore, when WBPL ended in 2001, its legacy was not only case reduction and morbidity reduction but also the promise of a range of new tools.

The strength of RNAS$^+$ is its role as research incubator, as shown by the continued development of transmission-blocking initiatives, such as artemether for schistosomiasis (Xiao, 2005), a domestic animal vaccine (Williams et al., 2019) and the drug tribendimidine with its broad-spectrum action against parasitic helminths including the FBTs (Panic et al., 2014).

Interestingly, by killing immature schistosomes, artemether has been shown to have a dual action as the immature schistosomula that are killed by the drug release antigens that raise immune responses preventing new infections (Bergquist et al., 2004). It is also interesting that the adult stages of the trematodes *S. mansoni*, *C. sinensis*, *F. hepatica* and *O. viverrini*, all found in the bile ducts or the veins in their definitive hosts, differ so much in their susceptibility to tribendimidine (Keiser et al., 2007) that this drug only holds promise for use against intestinal nematodes and the FBTs (Sayasone et al., 2018).

References

Bergquist, R., Utzinger, J., Chollet, J., Shu-Hua, X., Weiss, N.A., Tanner, M., 2004. Triggering of high-level resistance against Schistosoma mansoni reinfection by artemether in the mouse model. Am. J. Trop. Med. Hyg. 71 (6), 774–777.

Bergquist, R., Johansen, M.V., Utzinger, J., 2009. Diagnostic dilemmas in helminthology: what tools to use and when? Trends Parasitol 25 (4), 151–156.

Bergquist, R., Whittaker, M., 2012. Control of neglected tropical diseases in Asia Pacific: implications for health information priorities. Infect. Dis. Poverty 1 (1), 3. https://doi.org/10.1186/2049-9957-1-3.

Cai, P., Weerakoon, K.G., Mu, Y., Olveda, R.M., Ross, A.G., Olveda, D.U., McManus, D.P., 2019. Comparison of Kato Katz, antibody-based ELISA and droplet digital PCR diagnosis of schistosomiasis japonica: lessons learnt from a setting of low infection intensity. PLoS Negl. Trop. Dis. 13 (3), e0007228. https://doi.org/10.1371/journal.pntd.0007228. eCollection 2019 Mar.

Chen, J., Xu, J., Bergquist, R., Li, S.Z., Zhou, X.N., 2018. "Farewell to the god of plague": the importance of political commitment towards the elimination of schistosomiasis. Trop. Med. Infect. Dis. 3 (4), 108. https://doi.org/10.3390/tropicalmed3040108.

Chen, M.G., Feng, Z., 1999. Schistosomiasis control in China. Parasitol. Int. 48, 11–19.

Chen, M.G., 2005. Use of praziquantel for clinical treatment and morbidity control of schistosomiasis japonica in China: a review of 30 years' experience. Acta Trop. 96 (2-3), 168–176.

Dean, L., Njelesani, J., Mulamba, C., Dacombe, R., Mbabazi, P.S., Bates, I., 2018. Establishing an international laboratory network for neglected tropical diseases: understanding existing capacity in five WHO regions. Version 4. F1000Res. 7, 1464. https://doi.org/10.12688/f1000research.16196.4. eCollection 2018. (Study commissioned by the WHO Global Working Group on Capacity Strengthening for national NTD Programmes [APW200811893] which reports to the NTD Strategic Technical Advisory Group).

De-Jian, S., Xu-Li, D., Ji-Hui, D., 2013. The history of the elimination of lymphatic filariasis in China. Infect. Dis. Poverty 2 (1), 30. https://doi.org/10.1186/2049-9957-2-30.

Field, M.J., Gold, M.R., 1998. Summarizing Population Health: Directions for the Development and Application of Population Metrics. Institute of Medicine (US) Committee on Summary Measures of Population Health. National Academies Press (US), Washington (DC).

Heesterbeek, H., Anderson, R.M., Andreasen, V., Bansal, S., De Angelis, D., Dye, C., Eames, K.T., Edmunds, W.J., Frost, S.D., Funk, S., Hollingsworth, T.D., House, T., Isham, V., Klepac, P., Lessler, J., Lloyd-Smith, J.O., Metcalf, C.J., Mollison, D., Pellis, L., Pulliam, J.R., Roberts, M.G., Viboud, C., Isaac Newton Institute IDD Collaboration, 2015. Modeling infectious disease dynamics in the complex landscape of global health. Science 347 (6227). aaa4339. https://doi.org/10.1126/science.aaa4339.

Hägerstrand, T., 1970. What about people in regional science? Pap. Reg. Sci. Assoc. 24, 7–21.

Kato, T., Miura, M., 1954. On the comparison of some stool examination methods. Jpn. J. Parasitol. 3, 35.

Katz, N., Chaves, A., Pellegrino, J., 1972. A simple device for quantitative stool thick-smear technique in Schistosomiasis mansoni. Rev. Inst. Med. Trop. Sao Paulo 14, 397–400.

Khieu, V., Or, V., Tep, C., Odermatt, P., Tsuyuoka, R., Char, M.C., Brady, M.A., Sidwell, J., Yajima, A., Huy, R., Ramaiah, K.D., Muth, S., 2018. How elimination of lymphatic filariasis as a public health problem in the Kingdom of Cambodia was achieved. Infect. Dis. Poverty 7 (1), 15. https://doi.org/10.1186/s40249-018-0394-7.

Keiser, J., Shu-Hua, X., Chollet, J., Tanner, M., Utzinger, J., 2007. Evaluation of the in vivo activity of tribendimidine against Schistosoma mansoni, Fasciola hepatica, Clonorchis sinensis, and Opisthorchis viverrini. Antimicrob. Agents Chemother. 51 (3), 1096–1098. Epub 2006 Dec 28.

Li, Y.S., Kardorff, R., Richter, J., Sun, K.Y., Zhou, H., McManus, D.P., Hatz, C., 2004. Ultrasound organometry: the importance of body height adjusted normal ranges in assessing liver and spleen parameters among Chinese subjects with Schistosoma japonicum infection. Acta Trop. 92 (2), 133–138.

Maegraith, B., 1958. Schistosomiasis in China. Lancet 271, 208–214.

Malone, J.B., Bergquist, R., Rinaldi, L., 2016. Geospatial surveillance and response systems for schistosomiasis. In: James, B. (Ed.), Schistosoma: Biology, Pathology and Control. CRC Press, Boca Raton, FL, USA, pp. 479–497.

Malone, J.B., Bergquist, R., Martins, M., Luvall, J.C., 2019. Use of geospatial surveillance and response systems for vector-borne diseases in the elimination phase. Trop. Med. Infect. Dis. 4, 15–30, pii: E15.

Mao, S.P., Shao, B.R., 1982. Schistosomiasis control in the People's Republic of China. Am. J. Trop. Med. Hyg. 31, 92–99.

Murray, C.J., Ezzati, M., Flaxman, A.D., Lim, S., Lozano, R., Michaud, C., Naghavi, M., Salomon, J.A., Shibuya, K., Vos, T., Wikler, D., Lopez, A.D., 2012. GBD 2010: design, definitions, and metrics. Lancet 380 (9859), 2063–2066. https://doi.org/10.1016/S0140-6736(12)61899-6.

Neiger, B.L., Thackeray, R., Van Wagenen, S.A., Hanson, C.L., West, J.H., Barnes, M.D., Fagen, M.C., 2012. Use of social media in health promotion: purposes, key performance indicators, and evaluation metrics. Health Promot. Pract. 13 (2), 159–164. https://doi.org/10.1177/1524839911433467.

Nkengasong, J.N., Nsubuga, P., Nwanyanwu, O., Gershy-Damet, G.M., Roscigno, G., Bulterys, M., Schoub, B., KM, D.C., Birx, D., 2010. Laboratory systems and services are critical in global health: time to end the neglect? Am. J. Clin. Pathol. 134 (3), 368–373.

Olveda, R., Leonardo, L., Zheng, F., Sripa, B., Bergquist, R., Zhou, X.N., 2010. Coordinating research on neglected parasitic diseases in Southeast Asia through networking. Adv. Parasitol. 72, 55–77. https://doi.org/10.1016/S0065-308X(10)72003-0.

Olveda, R.M., Gray, D.J., 2019. Schistosomiasis in the Philippines: innovative control approach is needed if elimination is the goal. Trop. Med. Infect. Dis. 4 (2), 66–70. pii: E66. https://doi.org/10.3390/tropicalmed4020066.

Panic, G., Duthaler, U., Speich, B., Keiser, J., 2014. Repurposing drugs for the treatment and control of helminth infections. Int. J. Parasitol. Drugs Drug Resist. 4 (3), 185–200.

Qin, L.Z., Xu, J., Feng, T., Lv, S., Qian, Y.J., Zhang, L.J., Li, Y.L., Lv, C., Bergquist, R., Li, S.Z., Zhou, X.N., 2018. Field evaluation of a loop-mediated isothermal amplification (LAMP) platform for the detection of *Schistosoma japonicum* infection in *Oncomelania hupensis* snails. Trop. Med. Infect. Dis. 3 (4), 124–133. pii: E124. https://doi.org/10.3390/tropicalmed3040124.

Qiu, L.Z., Xue, H.C., 1990. Experimental diagnosis. In: Mao, S.P. (Ed.), Schistosome Biology and Control of Schistosomiasis. Publishing House for People's Health, Beijing, pp. 448–527. (in Chinese).

Ren, H.N., Cheng, B.Z., Zhuang, Z.N., 1987. Experimental therapeutic efficacy of a new anti-hookworm drug, tribendimidin. Zhongguo Ji Sheng Chong Xue Yu Ji Sheng Chong Bing Za Zhi 5, 262–264.

Rinaldi, L., Genchi, C., Musella, V., Genchi, M., Cringoli, G., 2011. Geographical information systems as a tool in the control of heartworm infections in dogs and cats. Vet. Parasitol. 176, 286–290.

Sayasone, S., Keiser, J., Meister, I., Vonghachack, Y., Xayavong, S., Senggnam, K., Phongluxa, K., Hattendorf, J., Odermatt, P., 2018. Efficacy and safety of tribendimidine versus praziquantel against Opisthorchis viverrini in Laos: an open-label, randomised, non-inferiority, phase 2 trial. Lancet Infect. Dis. 18 (2), 155–161. https://doi.org/10.1016/S1473-3099(17)30624-2. Epub 2017 Nov 16.

Stensgaard, A.S., Saarnak, C.F., Utzinger, J., Vounatsou, P., Simoonga, C., Mushinge, G., Rahbek, C., Møhlenberg, F., Kristensen, T.K., 2009. Virtual globes and geospatial health: the potential of new tools in the management and control of vector-borne diseases. Geospat. Health 3, 127–141.

Twardzik, E., Antonakos, C., Baiers, R., Dubowitz, T., Clarke, P., Colabianchi, N., 2018. Validity of environmental audits using GigaPan® and Google Earth Technology. Int. J. Health Geogr. 17, 26.

United Nations, 2015. The Agenda for Sustainable Development. https://sustainable development.un.org/?menu=1300. [(Accessed 28 June 2019)].

Utzinger, J., Zhou, X.N., Chen, M.G., Bergquist, R., 2005. Conquering schistosomiasis in China: the long march. Acta Trop. 96 (2-3), 69–96.

van Dam, G.J., Odermatt, P., Acosta, L., Bergquist, R., de Dood, C.J., Kornelis, D., Muth, S., Utzinger, J., Corstjens, P.L., 2015. Evaluation of banked urine samples for the detection of circulating anodic and cathodic antigens in Schistosoma mekongi and S. japonicum infections: a proof-of-concept study. Acta Trop. 141 (Pt B), 198–203.

Weerakoon, K.G., Gordon, C.A., McManus, D.P., 2018. DNA diagnostics for schistosomiasis control. Trop. Med. Infect. Dis. (3), 81–100. pii: E81. https://doi.org/10.3390/tropicalmed3030081. Review.

WHO, 2012. Accelerating work to overcome the global impact of neglected tropical diseases: a road map for implementation. In: Executive Summary https://apps.who.int/iris/bitstream/handle/10665/70809/WHO_HTM_NTD_2012.1_eng.pdf;jsessionid=736DE3DA2D8041A2A122BFCF5B2D5E04?sequence=1. accessed June 28 2019.

Williams, G.M., Li, Y.S., Gray, D.J., Zhao, Z.Y., Harn, D.A., Shollenberger, L.M., Li, S.M., Yu, X., Feng, Z., Guo, J.G., Zhou, J., Dong, Y.L., Li, Y., Guo, B., Driguez, P., Harvie, M., You, H., Ross, A.G., McManus, D.P., 2019. Field testing integrated interventions for schistosomiasis elimination in the People's Republic of China: outcomes of a multifactorial cluster-randomized controlled trial. Front. Immunol. 10, 645. https://doi.org/10.3389/fimmu.2019.00645. eCollection 2019.

Xiao, S.H., 2005. Development of antischistosomal drugs in China, with particular consideration to praziquantel and the artemisinins. Acta Trop. 96 (2–3), 153–167. Epub 2005 Aug 19. Review.

Yin, J.H., Yang, M.N., Zhou, S.S., Wang, Y., Feng, J., Xia, Z.G., 2013. Changing malaria transmission and implications in China towards National Malaria Elimination Programme between 2010 and 2012. PLoS One 8 (9), e74228. eCollection 2013. https://doi.org/10.1371/journal.pone.0074228.

Yu, J.M., de Vlas, S.J., Yuan, H.C., Gryseels, B., 1998. Variations in fecal *Schistosoma japonicum* egg counts. Am. J. Trop. Med. Hyg. 59 (3), 370–375.

Zhang, Z., Zhu, R., Ward, M.P., Xu, W., Zhang, L., Guo, J., Zhao, F., Jiang, Q., 2012. Long-term impact of the World Bank Loan Project for schistosomiasis control: a comparison of the spatial distribution of schistosomiasis risk in China. PLoS. Negl. Trop. Dis. 6 (4), e1620.

Zhou, X.N., Ohta, N., Utzinger, J., Bergquist, R., Olveda, R.M., 2008. RNAS(+): a win-win collaboration to combat neglected tropical diseases in Southeast Asia. Parasitol. Int. 57 (3), 243–245. https://doi.org/10.1016/j.parint.2008.04.001.

Zhu, H., Xu, J., Zhu, R., Cao, C., Bao, Z., Yu, Q., 2014. Comparison of the miracidium hatching test and modified Kato-Katz method for detecting *Schistosoma japonicum* in low prevalence areas of China. Southeast Asian J. Trop. Med. Public Health 45, 20–25.

Zhu, Y., He, W., Liang, Y., Xu, M., Yu, C., Hua, W., Chao, G., 2002. Development of a rapid, simple dipstick dye immunoassay for schistosomiasis diagnosis. J. Immunol. Methods 266 (1-2), 1–5.

Zhu, Y.C., Socheat, D., Bounlu, K., Liang, Y.S., Sinuon, M., Insisiengmay, S., He, W., Xu, M., Shi, W.Z., Bergquist, R., 2005. Application of dipstick dye immunoassay (DDIA) kit for the diagnosis of Schistosomiasis mekongi. Acta Trop. 96 (2-3), 137–141.

CHAPTER SEVEN

Challenges and way forward

Lydia Leonardo[a,*], Robert Bergquist[b], Juerg Utzinger[c], Shi-Zhu Li[d,e,f,g,h], Marilu Venturina[i], Xiao-Nong Zhou[d,e,f,g,h]

[a]Institute of Biology, College of Science, University of the Philippines Diliman and University of the East Ramon Magsaysay Graduate School, Quezon City, Philippines
[b]Geospatial Health, Ingerod, Brastad, Sweden
[c]Swiss Tropical and Public Health Institute, Basel, Switzerland
[d]National Institute of Parasitic Diseases, Chinese Center for Disease Control and Prevention, Shanghai, China
[e]Chinese Center for Tropical Diseases Research, Shanghai, China
[f]WHO Collaborating Centre for Tropical Diseases, Shanghai, China
[g]National Center for International Research on Tropical Diseases, Shanghai, China
[h]Key Laboratory of Parasite and Vector Biology, Ministry of Health, Shanghai, China
[i]Asian Tropical Foundation, Filinvest Corporate City, Research Institute for Tropical Medicine Compound, Muntinlupa, Philippines
*Corresponding author: e-mail address: lydialeonardo1152@gmail.com

Contents

1. Introduction 125
  1.1 Gaps in the research, control of schistosomiasis and other RNAS$^+$ target diseases 126
  1.2 Gaps possibly in the structure and operation of RNAS$^+$ 128
2. Way forward 130
References 132

Abstract

Schistosomiasis, helminthic zoonoses and NTDs constitute a considerable majority of the diseases of poverty in the world. The RNAS$^+$ targeted zoonoses are not only problems to human and animal health, but also cause poverty in 1 billion poor livestock keepers as well as result in 2.3 billion cases of human illness and 1.7 million human deaths a year. The gaps in research of those targeted zoonoses are urgently addressed by identifying the research priority, fulfilled by improving the multisectoral cooperation and strengthening the interventions in the control programme.

1. Introduction

Schistosomiasis, helminthic zoonoses and NTDs constitute a considerable majority of the diseases of poverty in the world. Discussions in annual RNAS$^+$ meetings stress the necessity of the socio-behavioural aspect of transmission of these diseases hence the advocacy for understanding affected

Advances in Parasitology, Volume 105
ISSN 0065-308X
https://doi.org/10.1016/bs.apar.2019.07.009

communities' knowledge, attitudes and practices to be able to formulate appropriate and acceptable strategies. Starting with the implementation of the EcoHealth approach, RNAS$^+$ continuously espouses the collaboration of various disciplines such as Veterinary Public Health, Sanitation, Human Health, Social Sciences, Education, Economics and Agriculture for the successful research and control and eventual elimination of all its target diseases(Malone et al., 2010; Yang et al., 2010).

Zoonotic diseases are not only considered as one of major problems in public health and animal health, but also regarded as an obstacle in the pathway out of poverty for 1 billion poor livestock keepers. These diseases also cause 2.3 billion cases of human illness and 1.7 million human deaths a year. In this light, RNAS$^+$ continues to address these issues through researches, interdisciplinary training, and advocacy for collaboration and multisectoral cooperation using the RNAS$^+$ platform, it is important to identify gaps in research and control for RNAS$^+$ targeted diseases to identify research priorities in future collaborative researches (Zhou et al., 2002, 2015).

1.1 Gaps in the research, control of schistosomiasis and other RNAS$^+$ target diseases

The RNAS$^+$ was founded mainly for the following objectives: (1) coordinate and secure support for research on surveillance and control of schistosomiasis transmission in humans and animals; (2) disseminate information about ongoing research and training activities; (3) develop standardized protocols for infection and disease surveillance; (4) evaluate current control strategies and assign regional research priorities; and (5) share plans for new studies and explore the potential for international collaboration (Zhou et al., 2008).

Its annual regular meetings were marked with presentations of research results on various aspects of schistosomiasis and other helminthic zoonoses such as clonorchiasis, opisthorchiasis, fascioliasis, paragonimiasis and taeniasis/cysticercosis and in more recent years also of NTDs such as lymphatic filariasis, soil-transmitted helminthiases, and food-borne trematodiases. In the last 20 years of RNAS$^+$, great progress has been achieved in the control and prevention of schistosomiasis with significant number of endemic areas in China, Indonesia, the Philippines, Laos and Cambodia reaching near elimination levels. New research needs have been realized with this development such as the urgent demand for development of more sensitive diagnostic methods to be used in surveillance and monitoring of schistosomiasis in areas that have reached near-elimination levels (Charlier et al., 2018; Olveda et al., 2010).

Recognizing the limitation of preventive chemotherapy alone in achieving elimination, a response to the urgent call for multifaceted response that would target the animal reservoir hosts, the snail intermediate host and the environment that perpetuates transmission, took the form of the EcoHealth approach involving multidisciplinary and multisectoral components. Techniques for surveillance, monitoring and evaluation continue to be developed in order to achieve elimination successfully. Standardization of surveillance techniques and assessment of intervention strategies remain an urgent plea for $RNAS^+$ to respond to. GIS and RS have been proved to be powerful tools for surveillance and monitoring but guidelines are still needed for their specific applications in various settings.

Vaccine development remains a possible option for prevention of re-infection complementing traditional methods such as preventive chemotherapy, snail control, environmental sanitation and health education. Mathematical modelling is continuously explored to elucidate how these various intervention measures can contribute to achieve the goal of elimination given a specific setting.

In an intensely dynamic socio-ecological environment, both ongoing and future events of this nature pose imminent threats to possible spread of schistosomiasis to other nonendemic areas visibly offsetting the gains that have been accomplished in many endemic areas. The Three Gorges Dam in China is forecasted to exert a massive change that could trigger widespread economic, social, ecologic and health changes (Poulin, 2002). There have been repeated warnings on the possible conditions created by the dam that favour perpetuation of schistosomiasis especially survival, reproduction and spread of the *Oncomelania* snails. The possibility of increase in snail habitats is also predicted as a result of the implementation of the policy of antiflooding of "disrupting banks to catch up more water, returning crop land into wet land of lake, relocation of new towns to settle people in high land".

The large scale water resources developments underway in Lao PDR also cause concern for possible emergence of snail habitats for *Schistosomiasis mekongi* and other snail-borne trematodes. In China, there is a call for establishment of regional intersectoral collaboration among the agricultural, health and hydrological sectors in the Yangtze River valley of the People's Republic of China, in order to block expansion and spread of the disease after flooding events.

In the early years of $RNAS^+$, Dr. Arve Lee Willingham then with the Danish Bilharzhiasis Laboratory saw the value of stressing the impact of schistosomiasis on food security and agricultural output through its effect on farmers and fishermen and consequently on animal production and health. Dr. Willingham named three C's that are essential in surveillance and control of schistosomiasis viz. communication, cooperation and coordination.

The expansion of the scope of RNAS$^+$ target diseases to other helminthic zoonoses and NTDs also elucidated specific research needs in these diseases such as research on burden of disease to surface the importance of cancer-causing diseases such as clonorchiasis and opisthorchiasis. The success in elimination of lymphatic filariasis needs to be shared with other member countries for their guidance and reference. Report of schistosomiasis in Myanmar needs to be confirmed and further elucidated to forewarn other countries which might face the same risk of emergence of this disease.

The benefits of intersectoral collaboration are numerous starting with how sectors can avail of creative synergies and accomplish mutual results that could be impossible for them to accomplish on their own alone. Combined interests, resources and responsibility can result in more sustainable solutions for coping with risks. Collective actions of the various collaborating sectors can bring about more innovative approaches to the process of policy design, action planning, policy implementation and monitoring and evaluation (Turner et al., 2015; Zhou et al., 2002).

1.2 Gaps possibly in the structure and operation of RNAS$^+$

1.2.1 Funding problems

The initial meetings of RNAS$^+$ were funded by WHO/TDR. Subsequent meetings were supported by particular government agencies of host country and funds from ongoing multi-country projects from IDRC and Mekong Subregion Project. Suggestions to explore other sources of funds to maintain the operations of RNAS$^+$ especially its regular meetings have always been in the agenda of its annual meetings. Possible fund sources such as FAO, ADB, World Bank, IFAD (International Foundation for Agricultural Development) have been proposed including the use of a more aggressive marketing of the organization to be able to obtain grants for multicountry and multidisciplinary researches similar to the IDRC project. Other recommendations include integrating malaria and NTDs in RNAS$^+$ proposals; stressing poverty alleviation through control of infections diseases in proposals; conducting social marketing to understand what donors want and lastly organizing international symposia that would generate funds from registration fees.

1.2.2 Role of RNAS⁺

Dr. Feng Zheng, the first president of the network proposed the following nature of the RNAS$^+$: that the organization should be an open network, not a closed circle that will be tasked with (1) disseminating knowledge and available technological information for further development; (2) application of new advancement in control programmes; (3) consolidating the network to bring more scientists in; (4) promoting intersectoral, interregional, and international collaboration; and (5) converting knowledge into action (Zhou et al., 2002).

On the issue of how the mandate of the RNAS$^+$ is distinguished from that of government institutions, RNAS$^+$ is suggested to take a role as a hub for government and researches to link for better utilization of resources. Furthermore, the activities of RNAS which should be looked at as a service organization, are expected to always be in consultation with the national control programme of the concerned country. The network also continues to coordinate with WHO—WPRO and endeavours to help the Ministry or Department of Health of the member countries.

The network also serves as both an information group and advisory group that is dependent on expert committees for proposal and development of policies, guidelines on research standards, research thrusts and researchable areas among others.

1.2.3 Network consolidation and expansion

In one annual network meeting, representatives from member countries recognized the need to strengthen communication among scientists engaged in schistosomiasis research, the importance of regular information exchange as well as the sharing of technologies involving control and surveillance. Dr. Remigio Olveda, two-time president of the proposed that the network device a way to bring together all those who have worked on ultrasound so they can come up with answers related to standardization of the protocol using ultrasonography.

Dr. Kevin Palmer of WHO in 2005, referred to RNAS as the most active network being supported by WHO at present. He joined the other speakers in calling for changes in the seven-year old network such as expanding its vision, looking into other areas of training and recruiting younger researchers and new control people. He warned about the resurgence of the disease in China and the waning importance and priority given to the disease in the Philippines. He stressed the need to revise objectives of the network to make it stronger, attractive and interesting to donors.

Other suggestions to consolidate and expand the network included the following. Invitations to meetings should be extended to officials of international organizations such as WHO, FAO, ILRI and others. The linkage with the RNAS$^+$ African counterpart should be revived and intensified.

Dr. Banchob Sripa of Thailand who served as president of RNAS$^+$ previously encouraged more communication with member countries through an improved website or even a Facebook account. This is also a way of gaining more visibility for the network. It was stressed that there is a need for suggestions and comments on how to improve the annual meetings.

There was a move to organize an email group to continue discussion among members about issues like surveillance, criteria for elimination and others, problems in MDA and other challenges encountered by member countries in the control and elimination of NTDs. Dr. Bergquist, one of the international advisors will moderate the group discussion on line and Dr. Lydia Leonardo, RNAS$^+$ secretary will document the discussion.

1.2.4 Research in RNAS$^+$ and training

RNAS$^+$ has undertaken multicountry and multidisciplinary researches in the past that contributed to advances in the knowledge about its target diseases leading to improvements in control. Increasing globalization and climate change that negatively impact the health, economy and socio-cultural aspects not only of RNAS$^+$ member countries but of the world in general necessitate research to mitigate the profound effects of these two global changes.

Collaborative researches and training courses are urgently called for since the network has constantly been in the forefront of research, information dissemination and translation of results for improvement of particular health programmes.

In anticipation of the changing of guards soon, a development plan should be made for the young scientists in the organization in terms of training for research proposal writing, research implementation and manuscript writing. They should also be assisted in the publication of papers in peer-reviewed journals.

2. Way forward

The search for funds will definitely be at top priority of the network as it marches into its third decade of existence. Strategies like expansion of target diseases, inclusion of more members and advocacy for multi-disease and more integrated interventions are expected to enhance its competitive ability. Annual meetings might not be enough to discuss and develop strategies to address this critical problem. Constant communication and discussion using available communication technologies might be needed to track down funding sources and prepare requirements needed for funding proposals.

$RNAS^+$ will continue to contribute to the reduction of disease burdens due to schistosomiasis and other NTDs through training, research and information dissemination. Focus will be on (i) improving the research environment through standardization of technologies, procedures and protocols used in prevention and control;(ii) facilitating dissemination of reliable and up-to-date information about Asian helminth zoonotic infections including the production of risk maps for the target diseases; and (iii) developing a surveillance and response system for the diseases that are approaching the elimination goal.

More focus will be directed at training activities in specific fields such as immunodiagnostics, standardization of ultrasound use for monitoring infection-related morbidity, cost factor analysis, application of GIS/RS technology, environmental modification and human behaviour, agricultural efforts including livestock management for control of schistosome transmission for all the target diseases of $RNAS^+$.

Priorities will remain on documentation and development of health metrics that are not only useful in practice, but also support research on the impact of social determinants and economic issues on the epidemiology of Asian helminth zoonotic infections and NTDs. To promote these priorities, important activities include the promotion of GIS and remote-sensing techniques for the study of climate change and direct, epidemiological applications, development of new products, equipment and techniques to improve and standardize diagnostic capabilities, and implementation research related to control strategies. Vaccine development will be pursued and enhanced through the study of genetics and the immune responses against parasites to better understand the pathology caused (Charlier et al., 2018; Olveda et al., 2010; Poulin, 2002; Turner et al., 2015).

Available mechanisms for information-sharing will remain in place such as the network framework, the website, databases, publications and meetings. Future emphasis will focus on platform design and technical standardization aiming at fostering strengthened research capacity and the development of networking capacities and easy access to information.

The coming years may or may not be tough on the network and definitely $RNAS^+$ will rely heavily on the strengths that is has developed in the past 20 years. These include its expertise such as in diagnostics, vaccine development, GIS and control strategies. It has a legal framework for networking and capacity to develop training packages such as for GIS, diagnosis, health metrics (e.g., burden assessment), molecular biology, vaccine and others. Its available mechanisms for sharing of information include a website, database, publications and regular meetings. It has a capacity to develop multidisciplinary approach, multicountry proposals for disease control. It has a direct linkage with different academic and research institutions competitive advantage as well as a strong linkage with control programmes of endemic member countries.

Challenges and opportunities will remain and will change in the forthcoming years and the survival of the network will depend on how well it will utilize its strengths as well as develop the next batch of leaders and members who will be at the frontline.

References

Charlier, J., Thamsborg, S.M., Bartley, D.J., Skuce, P.J., Kenyon, F., Geurden, T., Hoste, H., Williams, A.R., Sotiraki, S., Hoglund, J., Chartier, C., Geldhof, P., van Dijk, J., Rinaldi, L., Morgan, E.R., von Samson-Himmelstjerna, G., Vercruysse, J., Claerebout, E., 2018. Mind the gaps in research on the control of gastrointestinal nematodes of farmed ruminants and pigs. Transbound. Emerg. Dis. 65 (Suppl. 1), 217–234.

Malone, J.B., Yang, G.J., Leonardo, L., Zhou, X.N., 2010. Implementing a geospatial health data infrastructure for control of Asian schistosomiasis in the People's Republic of China and the Philippines. Adv. Parasitol. 73, 71–100.

Olveda, R., Leonardo, L., Zheng, F., Sripa, B., Bergquist, R., Zhou, X.N., 2010. Coordinating research on neglected parasitic diseases in Southeast Asia through networking. Adv. Parasitol. 72, 55–77.

Poulin, R., 2002. Qualitative and quantitative aspects of recent research on helminth parasites. J. Helminthol. 76 (4), 373–376.

Turner, H.C., Truscott, J.E., Hollingsworth, T.D., Bettis, A.A., Brooker, S.J., Anderson, R.M., 2015. Cost and cost-effectiveness of soil-transmitted helminth treatment programmes: systematic review and research needs. Parasit. Vectors 8, 355.

Yang, G.J., Utzinger, J., Lv, S., Qian, Y.J., Li, S.Z., Wang, Q., Bergquist, R., Vounatsou, P., Li, W., Yang, K., Zhou, X.N., 2010. The Regional Network for Asian schistosomiasis and Other Helminth Zoonoses (RNAS(+)) target diseases in face of climate change. Adv. Parasitol. 73, 101–135.

Zhou, X., Acosta, L., Willingham 3rd, A.L., Leonardo, L.R., Minggang, C., Aligui, G., Zheng, F., Olveda, R., 2002. Regional Network for research, surveillance and control of Asian schistosomiasis (RNAS). Acta Trop. 82 (2), 305–311.

Zhou, X.N., Ohta, N., Utzinger, J., Bergquist, R., Olveda, R.M., 2008. RNAS(+): a win-win collaboration to combat neglected tropical diseases in Southeast Asia. Parasitol. Int. 57 (3), 243–245.

Zhou, X.N., Olveda, R., Sripa, B., Yang, G.J., Leonardo, L., Bergquist, R., 2015. From gap analysis to solution and action: the RNAS(+) model. Acta Trop. 141 (Pt. B), 146–149.

Annex 1: Publications through RNAS$^+$ platform

Marilu O. Venturina[a], Lydia Leonardo[b], Robert Bergquist[c], Xiao-Nong Zhou[d,e,f,g,h]

[a]Asian Tropical Foundation, Filinvest Corporate City, Research Institute for Tropical Medicine Compound, Alabang, Muntinlupa, Philippines
[b]Institute of Biology, College of Science, University of the Philippines Diliman and University of the East Ramon Magsaysay Graduate School, Philippines
[c]Geospatial Health, Ingerod, Brastad, Sweden
[d]National Institute of Parasitic Diseases, Chinese Center for Disease Control and Prevention, Shanghai, China
[e]Chinese Center for Tropical Diseases Research, Shanghai, China
[f]WHO Collaborating Centre for Tropical Diseases, Shanghai, China
[g]National Center for International Research on Tropical Diseases, Shanghai, China
[h]Key Laboratory of Parasite and Vector Biology, Ministry of Health, Shanghai, China

During last 20 years, more than 20 articles were published to record all activities and research outcomes under platform of RNAS$^+$, by investigators, coordinators, and partners. We present herewith all references of those publications, in order to easily understand the evolution ways of RNAS$^+$ development.

1. Song, L.G., Zeng, X.D., Li, Y.X., Zhang, B.B., Wu, X.Y., Yuan, D.J., He, A., Wu, Z.D., 2018. Imported parasitic diseases in mainland China: current status and perspectives for better control and prevention. Infect Dis Poverty 7, 78.
2. Tambo, E., Ai, L., Zhou, X., Chen, J.H., Hu, W., Bergquist, R., Guo, J.G., Utzinger, J., Tanner, M., Zhou, X.N., 2014. Surveillance-response systems: the key to elimination of tropical diseases. Infect Dis Poverty 3, 17.
3. van Dam, G.J., Odermatt, P., Acosta, L., Bergquist, R., de Dood, C.J., Kornelis, D., Muth, S., Utzinger, J., Corstjens, P.L., 2015. Evaluation of banked urine samples for the detection of circulating anodic and cathodic antigens in Schistosoma mekongi and S. japonicum infections: a proof-of-concept study. Acta Trop 141, 198-203.
4. Weerakoon, K.G., Gordon, C.A., Williams, G.M., Cai, P., Gobert, G. N., Olveda, R.M., Ross, A.G., Olveda, D.U., McManus, D.P., 2018. Co-parasitism of intestinal protozoa and Schistosoma japonicum in a rural community in the Philippines. Infect Dis Poverty 7, 121.
5. Xiao, S.H., Sun, J., Chen, M.G., 2018. Pharmacological and immunological effects of praziquantel against Schistosoma japonicum: a scoping review of experimental studies. Infect Dis Poverty 7, 9.

6. Xu, J., Bergquist, R., Qian, Y.J., Wang, Q., Yu, Q., Peeling, R., Croft, S., Guo, J.G., Zhou, X.N., 2016. China-Africa and China-Asia Collaboration on Schistosomiasis Control: A SWOT Analysis. Adv Parasitol 92, 435-466.
7. Yang, X., Zhang, Y., Sun, Q.X., Zhou, J.X., Zhou, X.N., 2019. SWOT analysis on snail control measures applied in the national schistosomiasis control programme in the People's Republic of China. Infect Dis Poverty 8, 13.
8. Yin, M., Li, H., McManus, D.P., Blair, D., Su, J., Yang, Z., Xu, B., Feng, Z., Hu, W., 2015a. Geographical genetic structure of Schistosoma japonicum revealed by analysis of mitochondrial DNA and microsatellite markers. Parasit Vectors 8, 150.
9. Yin, M., Zheng, H.X., Su, J., Feng, Z., McManus, D.P., Zhou, X.N., Jin, L., Hu, W., 2015b. Co-dispersal of the blood fluke Schistosoma japonicum and Homo sapiens in the Neolithic Age. Sci Rep 5, 18058.
10. You, H., Cai, P., Tebeje, B.M., Li, Y., McManus, D.P., 2018. Schistosome Vaccines for Domestic Animals. Trop Med Infect Dis 3.
11. Young, N.D., Chan, K.G., Korhonen, P.K., Min Chong, T., Ee, R., Mohandas, N., Koehler, A.V., Lim, Y.L., Hofmann, A., Jex, A.R., Qian, B., Chilton, N.B., Gobert, G.N., McManus, D.P., Tan, P., Webster, B.L., Rollinson, D., Gasser, R.B., 2015. Exploring molecular variation in Schistosoma japonicum in China. Sci Rep 5, 17345.
12. Zhou, X., Acosta, L., Willingham, A.L., 3rd, Leonardo, L.R., Minggang, C., Aligui, G., Zheng, F., Olveda, R., 2002. Regional Network for Research, Surveillance and Control of Asian Schistosomiasis (RNAS). Acta Trop 82, 305-311.
13. Zhou, X.N., Ohta, N., Utzinger, J., Bergquist, R., Olveda, R.M., 2008. RNAS(+): A win-win collaboration to combat neglected tropical diseases in Southeast Asia. Parasitol Int 57, 243-245.
14. Zhou, X.N., Olveda, R., Sripa, B., Yang, G.J., Leonardo, L., Bergquist, R., 2015. From gap analysis to solution and action: the RNAS(+) model. Acta Trop 141, 146-149.
15. Attwood, S.W., Ibaraki, M., Saitoh, Y., Nihei, N., Janies, D.A., 2015. Comparative Phylogenetic Studies on Schistosoma japonicum and Its Snail Intermediate Host Oncomelania hupensis: Origins, Dispersal and Coevolution. PLoS Negl Trop Dis 9, e0003935.
16. Bergquist, R., Elmorshedy, H., 2018. Artemether and Praziquantel: Origin, Mode of Action, Impact, and Suggested Application for Effective Control of Human Schistosomiasis. Trop Med Infect Dis 3.

17. Cai, P., Weerakoon, K.G., Mu, Y., Olveda, R.M., Ross, A.G., Olveda, D.U., McManus, D.P., 2019. Comparison of Kato Katz, antibody-based ELISA and droplet digital PCR diagnosis of schistosomiasis japonica: Lessons learnt from a setting of low infection intensity. PLoS Negl Trop Dis 13, e0007228.

18. Dong, Y., Du, C.H., Zhang, Y., Wang, L.F., Song, J., Wu, M.S., Yang, W.C., Lv, S., Zhou, X.N., 2018. Role of ecological approaches to eliminating schistosomiasis in Eryuan County evaluated by system modelling. Infect Dis Poverty 7, 129.

19. Gordon, C.A., Kurscheid, J., Williams, G.M., Clements, A.C.A., Li, Y., Zhou, X.N., Utzinger, J., McManus, D.P., Gray, D.J., 2019. Asian Schistosomiasis: Current Status and Prospects for Control Leading to Elimination. Trop Med Infect Dis 4.

20. Ito, A., Li, T., Chen, X., Long, C., Yanagida, T., Nakao, M., Sako, Y., Okamoto, M., Wu, Y., Raoul, F., Giraudoux, P., Craig, P.S., 2013. Mini review on chemotherapy of taeniasis and cysticercosis due to Taenia solium in Asia, and a case report with 20 tapeworms in China. Trop Biomed 30, 164-173.

21. Kongklieng, A., Kaewkong, W., Intapan, P.M., Sanpool, O., Janwan, P., Thanchomnang, T., Lulitanond, V., Sri-Aroon, P., Limpanont, Y., Maleewong, W., 2013. Molecular differentiation of Schistosoma japonicum and Schistosoma mekongi by real-time PCR with high resolution melting analysis. Korean J Parasitol 51, 651-656.

22. Li, J., Chen, F., Sugiyama, H., Blair, D., Lin, R.Q., Zhu, X.Q., 2015. A specific indel marker for the Philippines Schistosoma japonicum revealed by analysis of mitochondrial genome sequences. Parasitol Res 114, 2697-2704.

23. Liang, S., Abe, E.M., Zhou, X.N., 2018. Integrating ecological approaches to interrupt schistosomiasis transmission: opportunities and challenges. Infect Dis Poverty 7, 124.

24. Liu, L., Huo, G.N., He, H.B., Zhou, B., Attwood, S.W., 2014. A phylogeny for the pomatiopsidae (Gastropoda: Rissooidea): a resource for taxonomic, parasitological and biodiversity studies. BMC Evol Biol 14, 29.

25. Lovis, L., Mak, T.K., Phongluxa, K., Aye Soukhathammavong, P., Vonghachack, Y., Keiser, J., Vounatsou, P., Tanner, M., Hatz, C., Utzinger, J., Odermatt, P., Akkhavong, K., 2012. Efficacy of praziquantel against Schistosoma mekongi and Opisthorchis viverrini: a randomized, single-blinded dose-comparison trial. PLoS Negl Trop Dis 6, e1726.

26. Lu, X.T., Gu, Q.Y., Limpanont, Y., Song, L.G., Wu, Z.D., Okanurak, K., Lv, Z.Y., 2018. Snail-borne parasitic diseases: an update on global epidemiological distribution, transmission interruption and control methods. Infect Dis Poverty 7, 28.

27. Lu, Y., Gonzales, G., Chen, S.H., Li, H., Cai, Y.C., Chu, Y.H., Ai, L., Chen, M.X., Chen, H.N., Chen, J.X., 2017. Urgent needs in fostering neglected tropical diseases (NTDs) laboratory capacity in WHO Western Pacific Region: results from the external quality assessment on NTDs diagnosis in 2012-2015. Infect Dis Poverty 6, 106.

28. Lv, S., Zhang, Y., Zhang, L., Liu, Q., Liu, H.X., Hu, L., Wei, F.R., Steinmann, P., Graeff-Teixeira, C., Zhou, X.N., Utzinger, J., 2012. The complete mitochondrial genome of the rodent intra-arterial nematodes Angiostrongylus cantonensis and Angiostrongylus costaricensis. Parasitol Res 111, 115-123.

29. Madsen, H., Hung, N.M., 2014. An overview of freshwater snails in Asia with main focus on Vietnam. Acta Trop 140, 105-117.

30. Madsen, H., Hung, N.M., 2015. Reprint of "An overview of freshwater snails in Asia with main focus on Vietnam". Acta Trop 141, 372-384.

31. Malone, J.B., Yang, G.J., Leonardo, L., Zhou, X.N., 2010. Implementing a geospatial health data infrastructure for control of Asian schistosomiasis in the People's Republic of China and the Philippines. Adv Parasitol 73, 71-100.

32. McManus, D.P., Dunne, D.W., Sacko, M., Utzinger, J., Vennervald, B.J., Zhou, X.N., 2018. Schistosomiasis. Nat Rev Dis Primers 4, 13.

33. Moendeg, K.J., Angeles, J.M.M., Nakao, R., Leonardo, L.R., Fontanilla, I.K.C., Goto, Y., Kirinoki, M., Villacorte, E.A., Rivera, P.T., Inoue, N., Chigusa, Y., Kawazu, S.I., 2017. Geographic strain differentiation of Schistosoma japonicum in the Philippines using microsatellite markers. PLoS Negl Trop Dis 11, e0005749.

34. Piratae, S., Tesana, S., Jones, M.K., Brindley, P.J., Loukas, A., Lovas, E., Eursitthichai, V., Sripa, B., Thanasuwan, S., Laha, T., 2012. Molecular characterization of a tetraspanin from the human liver fluke, Opisthorchis viverrini. PLoS Negl Trop Dis 6, e1939.

35. Willingham, A.L., Wu, H.W., Conlan, J., et al., 2010. Combating Taenia solium cysticercosis in Southeast Asia: an opportunity for improving human health and livestock production. Adv. Parasitol. 72, 235–266.

36. Zhou, X.N., Wayling, S., Bergquist, R., 2010. Concepts in research capabilities strengthening positive experiences of network approaches by TDR in the People's Republic of China and Eastern Asia. Adv. Parasitol. 73, 1–19.

37. Olveda, R., Leonardo, L., Zheng, F., et al., 2010. Coordinating research on neglected parasitic diseases in Southeast Asia through networking. Adv. Parasitol. 72, 55–77.
38. Hotez, P.J., Ehrenberg, J.P., 2010. Escalating the global fight against neglected tropical diseases through interventions in the Asia Pacific region-chapter 2. Adv. Parasitol. 72 (2), 31.
39. Zhou, X.N., Olveda, R., Sripa, B., et al., 2015. From gap analysis to solution and action: the RNAS$^+$ model. Acta Trop. 141 (Part B, Sp. Iss. SI), 146–149.
40. Hotez, P.J., Bottazzi, M.E., Strych, U., et al., 2015. Neglected tropical diseases among the Association of Southeast Asian Nations (ASEAN): overview and update. PLoS. Negl. Trop. Dis. 9 (4), e0003575.
41. Zhou, X., Acosta, L., Willingham, A.L., et al., 2002. Regional Network for Research, Surveillance and Control of Asian Schistosomiasis (RNAS). Acta Trop. 82 (2), 305–311.
42. Leonardo, L.R., Bergquist, R., 2002. Regional network on Asian schistosomiasis. Trends Parasitol. 18 (10), 434–436.
43. Yang, G.J., Utzinger, J., Lv, S., et al., 2010. The regional network for Asian schistosomiasis and other Helminth Zoonoses (RNAS$^+$): target diseases in face of climate change. Adv. Parasitol. 73, 101.
44. Li-Juan, Z., Jing, X., Lü S., et al., 2018. Development and role of Regional Network for Asian Schistosomiasis and other Helminth Zoonoses. Chin. J. Schistosomiasis Control 30 (1), 5–8.
45. Yang, G.J., Utzinger, J., Lv, S., et al., 2010. The Regional Network for Asian schistosomiasis and other Helminth Zoonoses (RNAS$^+$): target diseases in face of climate change. Adv. Parasitol. 73, 101.
46. Zhou, X., Acosta, L., Willingham, A.L., et al., 2002. Regional Network for Research, Surveillance and Control of Asian Schistosomiasis (RNAS). Acta Trop. 82 (2), 305–311.
47. Zhou, X.N., Bergquist, R., Leonardo, L., et al., 2012. Schistosomiasis japonica control and research needs. Adv. Parasitol. 72, 145.
48. Sripa, B., 2008. Concerted action is needed to tackle liver fluke infections in Asia. PLoS Negl. Trop. Dis. 2 (5), e232.
49. Leonardo, L.R., Bergquist, R., 2002. Regional network on Asian schistosomiasis. Trends Parasitol. 18 (10), 434–436.
50. Utzinger, J., Bergquist, R., Olveda, R., et al., 2010. Important Helminth infections in Southeast Asia: diversity, potential for control and prospects for elimination. Adv. Parasitol. 72 (C), 1–30.

51. Utzinger, J., Brattig, N.W., Leonardo, L., et al., 2015. Progress in research, control and elimination of Helminth infections in Asia. Acta Trop. 141(Pt B), 135–145.

52. Balen, J., 2007. Prevalence, intensity and associated morbidity of Schistosoma japonicum infection in the Dongting Lake region, China. Bull. World Health Organ., 85 (7), 519–526.

53. Leonardo, L.R., Acosta, L.P., Olveda, R.M., et al., 2002. Difficulties and strategies in the control of schistosomiasis in the Philippines. Acta Trop. 82 (2), 295–299.

54. Willingham, A.L., Wu, H.W., Conlan, J., et al., 2010. Combating Taenia solium cysticercosis in Southeast Asia: an opportunity for improving human health and livestock production. Adv. Parasitol. 72, 235–266.

55. Wu, X.H., Wang, X.H., Utzinger, Jürg, et al., 2007. Spatio-temporal correlation between human and bovine schistosomiasis in China: insight from three national sampling surveys. Geospat. Health. 2 (1), 75–84.

Annex 2: The memory photos in the selected RNAS$^+$ annual workshops

Marilu O. Venturina[a], Lydia Leonardo[b], Xiao-Nong Zhou[c,d,e,f,g]
[a]Asian Tropical Foundation, Filinvest Corporate City, Research Institute for Tropical Medicine Compound, Alabang, Muntinlupa, Philippines
[b]Institute of Biology, College of Science, University of the Philippines Diliman and University of the East Ramon Magsaysay Graduate School, Philippines
[c]National Institute of Parasitic Diseases, Chinese Center for Disease Control and Prevention, Shanghai, China
[d]Chinese Center for Tropical Diseases Research, Shanghai, China
[e]WHO Collaborating Centre for Tropical Diseases, Shanghai, China
[f]National Center for International Research on Tropical Diseases, Shanghai, China
[g]Key Laboratory of Parasite and Vector Biology, Ministry of Health, Shanghai, China

All most every annual workshop would take a family photo in order to memorize where and when the annual workshop was held. Therefore, we selected some of memory photos to attach in this special issue for our remembering those support and contribute to the development of RNAS$^+$ in the history.

1. The family photo in the 2nd RNAS workshop
2. The family photo in the 3rd RNAS workshop
3. The family photo in the 4th RNAS workshop
4. The family photo in the 7th RNAS workshop
5. The family photo in the 9th RNAS workshop
6. The family photo in the 12th RNAS workshop
7. The family photo in the 13th RNAS workshop
8. The family photo in the 13th RNAS workshop
9. The family photo in the 13th RNAS workshop
10. The family photo in the 14th RNAS workshop
11. The family photo in the 15th RNAS workshop
12. The family photo in the 17th RNAS workshop
13. The family photo in the 17th RNAS workshop

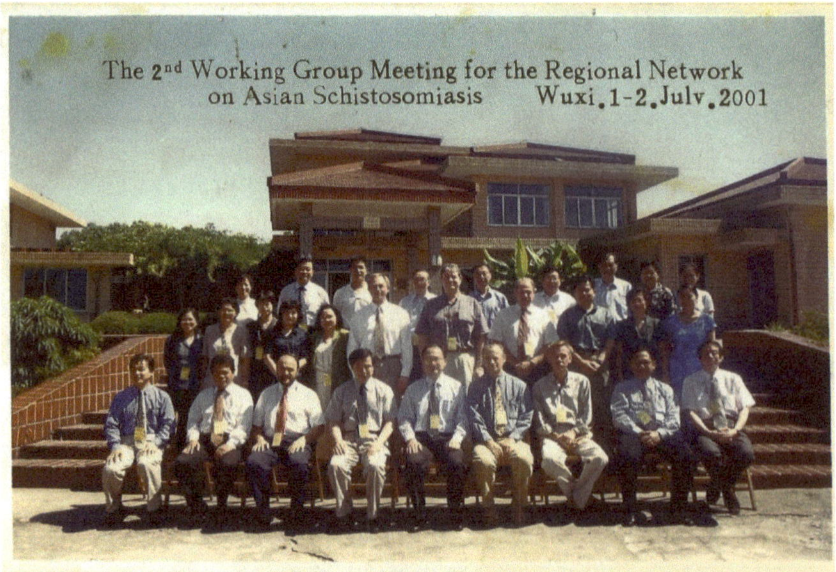
The 2nd Working Group Meeting for the Regional Network
on Asian Schistosomiasis Wuxi.1-2.July.2001

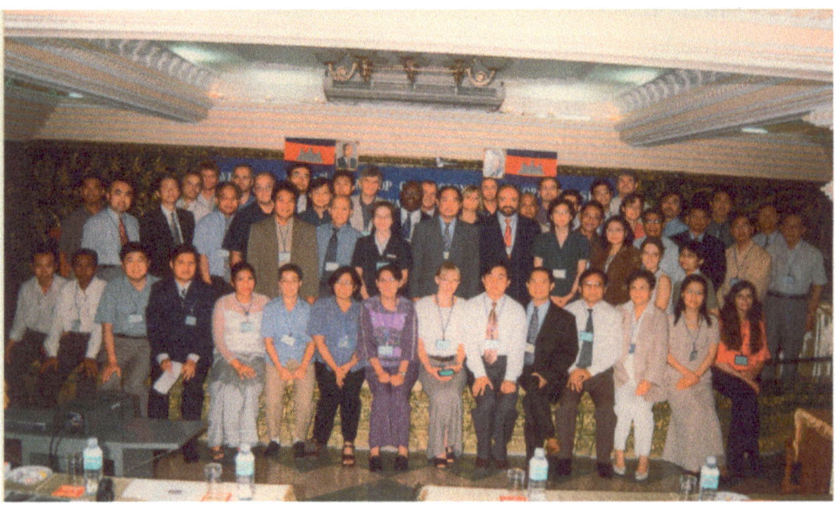

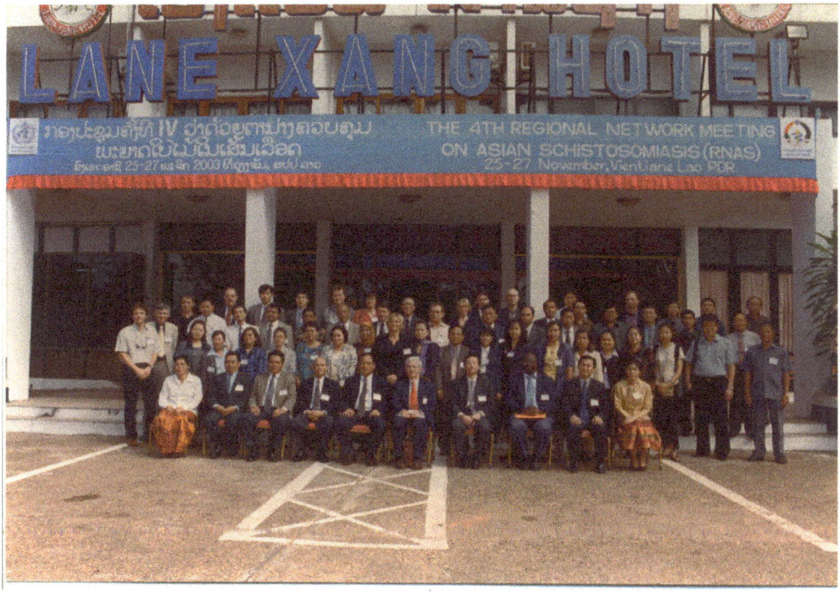
LANE XANG HOTEL
THE 4TH REGIONAL NETWORK MEETING
ON ASIAN SCHISTOSOMIASIS (RNAS)
25-27 November, Vientiane Lao PDR

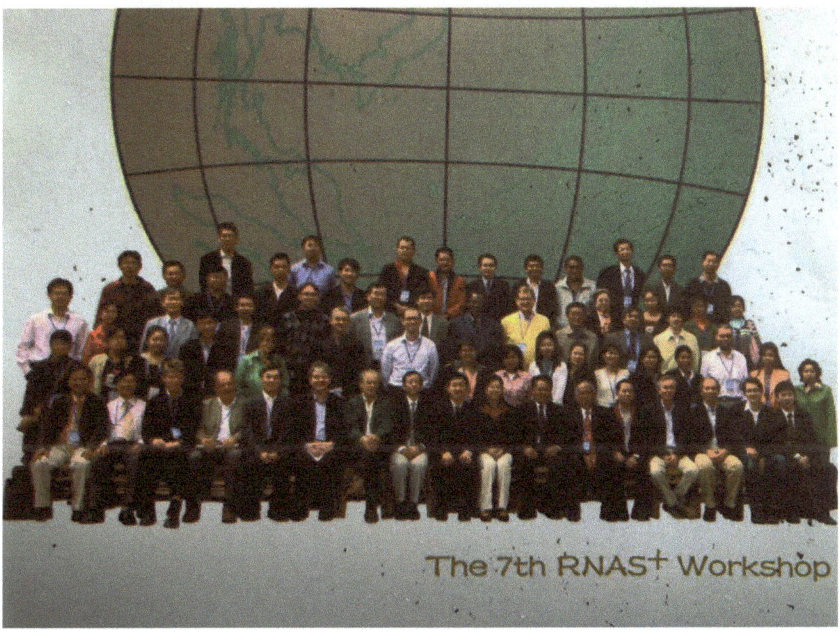
The 7th RNAS+ Workshop

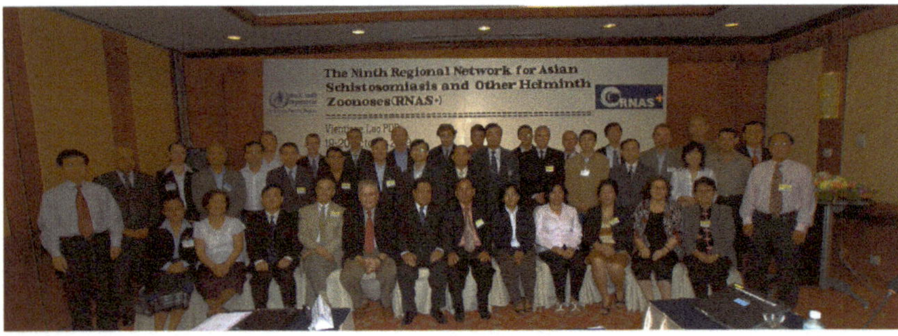
The Ninth Regional Network for Asian
Schistosomiasis and Other Helminth
Zoonoses(RNAS+)
RNAS+

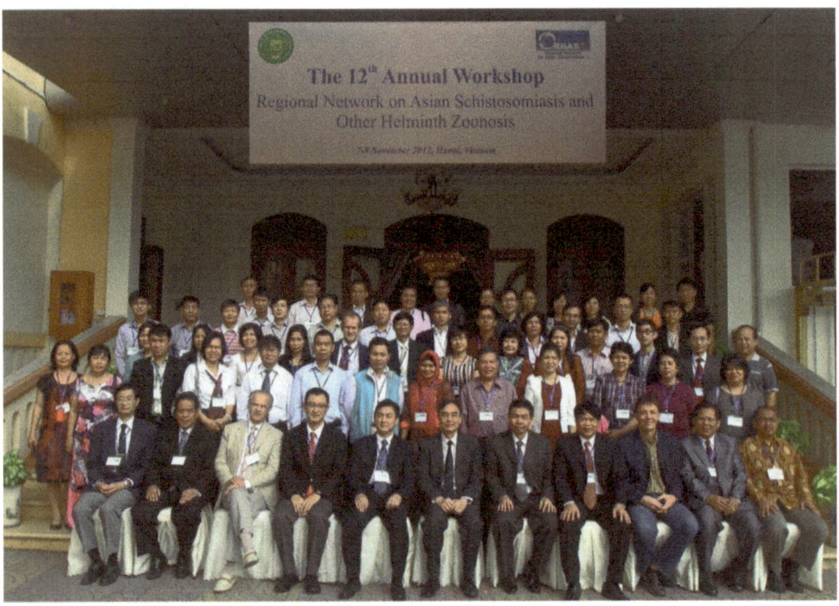
RNAS
The 12th Annual Workshop
Regional Network on Asian Schistosomiasis and
Other Helminth Zoonosis

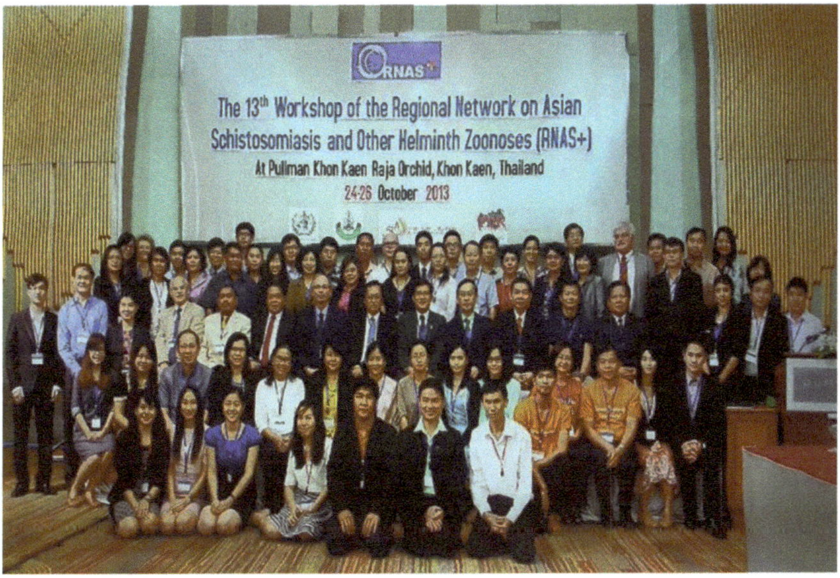
RNAS+
The 13th Workshop of the Regional Network on Asian
Schistosomiasis and Other Helminth Zoonoses (RNAS+)
At Pullman Khon Kaen Raja Orchid, Khon Kaen, Thailand
24-26 October 2013

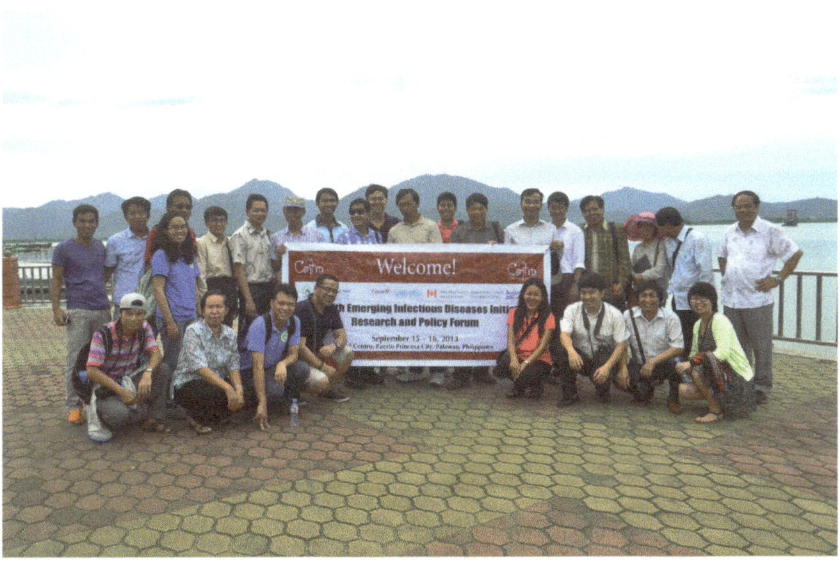
Welcome!
Research and Policy Forum

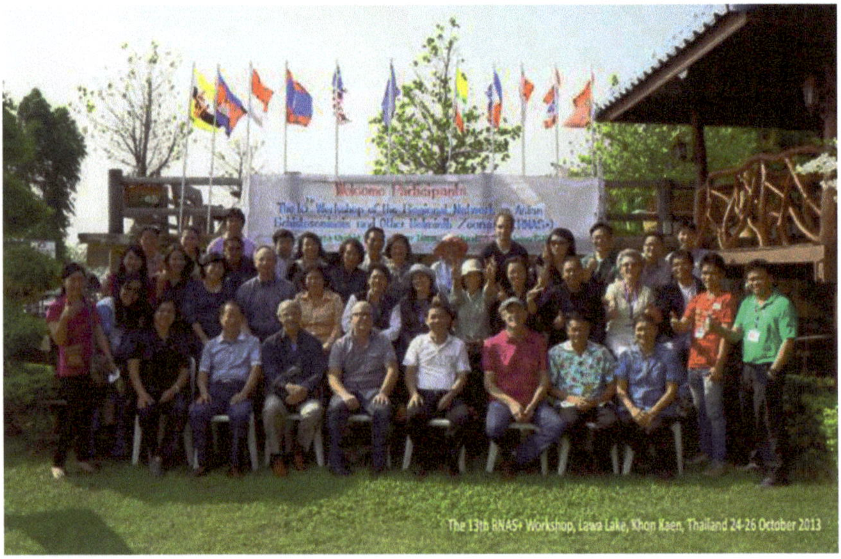
Welcome Participants
The 13th RNAS+ Workshop, Lawa Lake, Khon Kaen, Thailand 24-26 October 2013

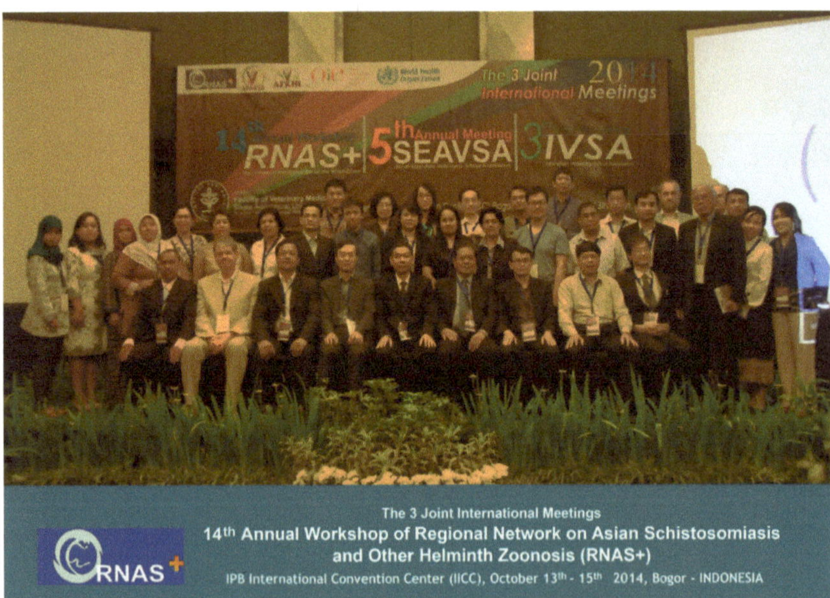
The 3 Joint International Meetings
2014
RNAS+
5th Annual Meeting SEAVSA
3 IVSA
RNAS+
The 3 Joint International Meetings
14th Annual Workshop of Regional Network on Asian Schistosomiasis and Other Helminth Zoonosis (RNAS+)
IPB International Convention Center (IICC), October 13th - 15th 2014, Bogor - INDONESIA

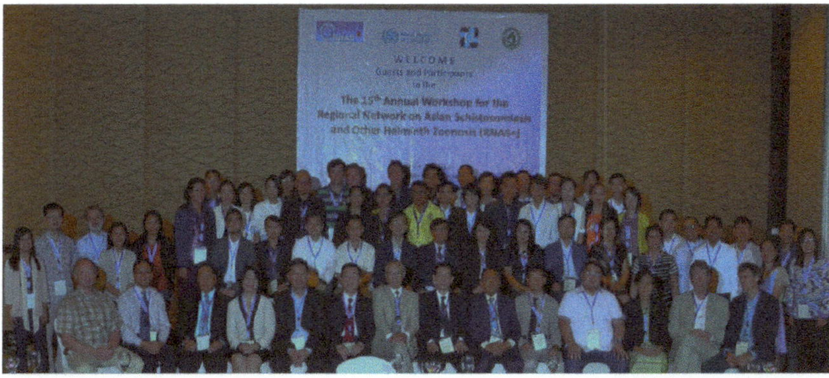
WELCOME
The 15th Annual Workshop for the
Regional Network on Asian Schistosomiasis
and Other Helminth Zoonosis (RNAS+)

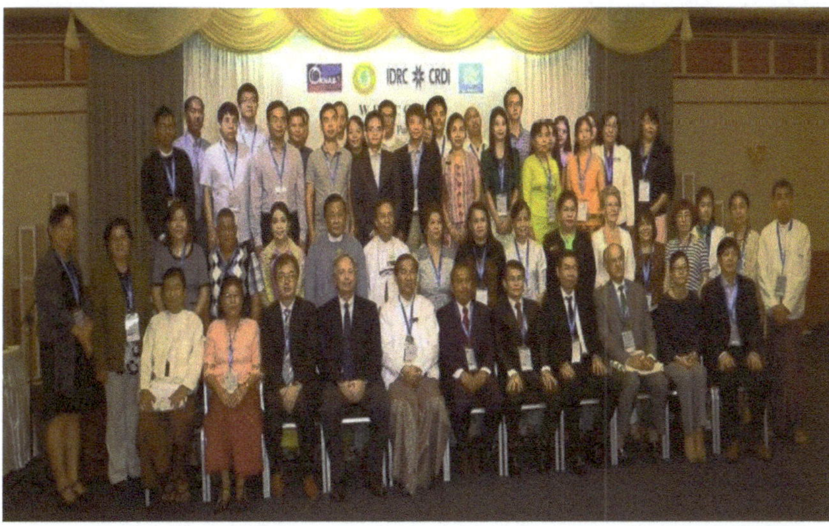
IDRC CRDI

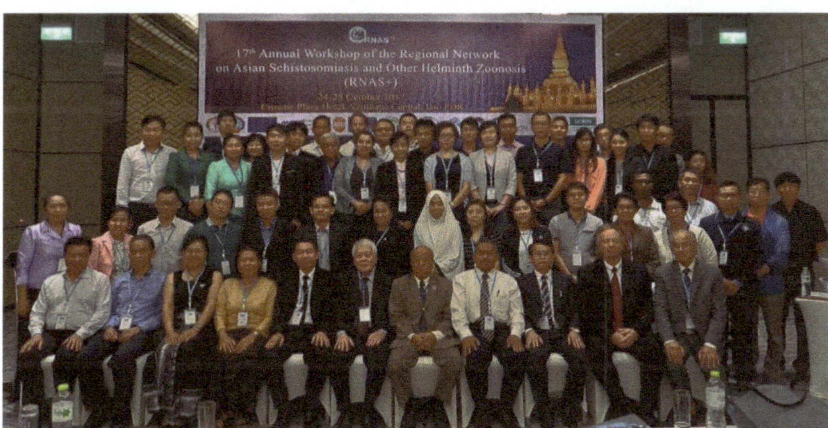
RNAS+
17th Annual Workshop of the Regional Network
on Asian Schistosomiasis and Other Helminth Zoonosis
(RNAS+)

Annex 3: Mapping the NTDs over RNAS$^+$ countries

Jin-Xin Zhen[a,b,c,d,e], Xiao-Nong Zhou[a,b,c,d,e]
[a]National Institute of Parasitic Diseases, Chinese Center for Disease Control and Prevention, Shanghai, China
[b]Chinese Center for Tropical Diseases Research, Shanghai, China
[c]WHO Collaborating Centre for Tropical Diseases, Shanghai, China
[d]National Center for International Research on Tropical Diseases, Shanghai, China
[e]Key Laboratory of Parasite and Vector Biology, Ministry of Health, Shanghai, China

1. NTDs Mapping

Neglected tropical diseases (NTDs)—a diverse group of communicable diseases that prevail in tropical and subtropical conditions in 149 countries—affect more than 1 billion people and cost developing economies billions of dollars every year. Populations living in poverty, without adequate sanitation and in close contact with infectious vectors and domestic animals and livestock are those worst affected. See https://www.who.int/neglected_diseases/diseases/en/.

Here we collect the public health of NTDs data from WHO, including *schistosomiasis*, *cysticercosis*, *clonorchiasis*, *opisthorchiasis*, *paragonimiasis* and *fascioliasis* in the following countries:

- Australia
- Cambodia
- China
- Indonesia
- Japan
- Lao PDR
- Malaysia
- Myanmar
- Philippine
- South Korea
- Thailand
- Vietnam

1.1 Schistosomiasis

Using the data from WHO https://www.who.int/schistosomiasis/en/ mapping the Population requiring PC for SCH annually data in 12 countries. Scaling from 1999 to 2018.

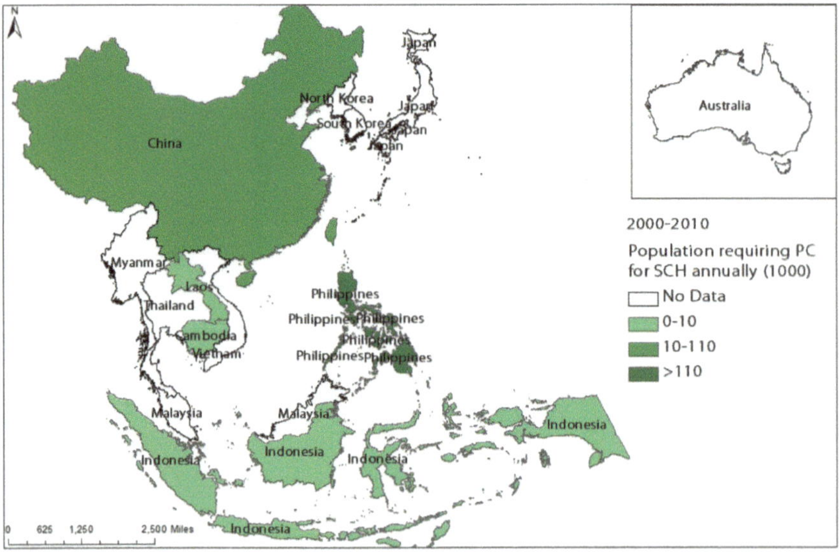

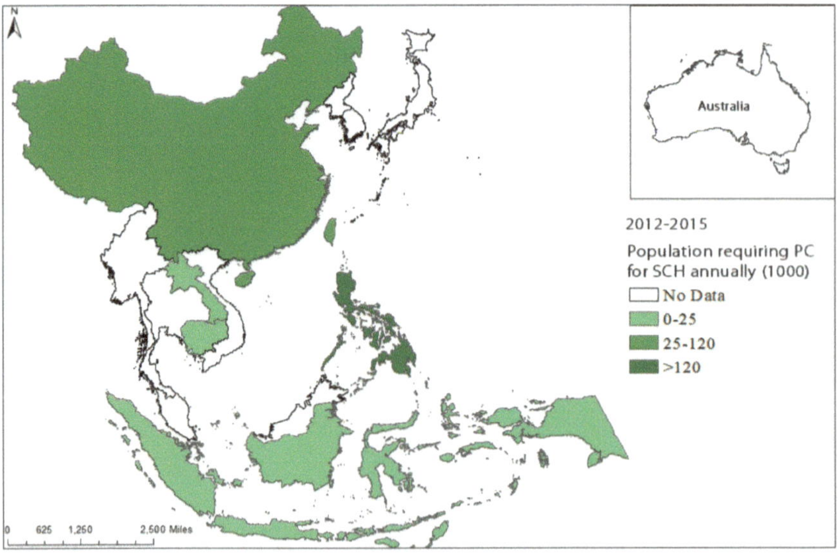

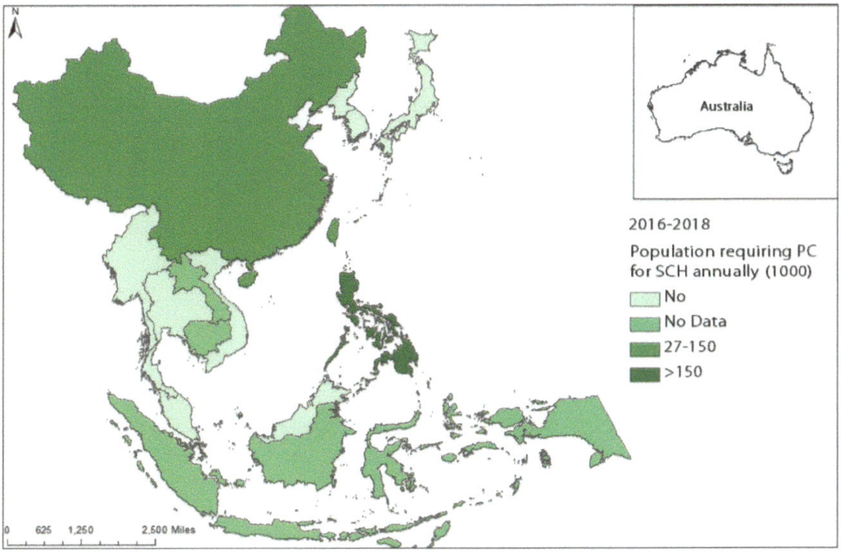

Most of countries are the endemic areas. The Philippine, Lao PDR, and Cambodia need to increase treatment in high transmission zones.

1.2 Cysticercosis

The map used by WHO to illustrate the endemicity of *T. solium* was updated in 2015, following a review of relevant literature and other indicators describing the likely transmission of the parasite, which from https://www.who.int/taeniasis/resources/who_wer914950b/en/.

From this map we only focus on the endemic areas, which are update to 2018.

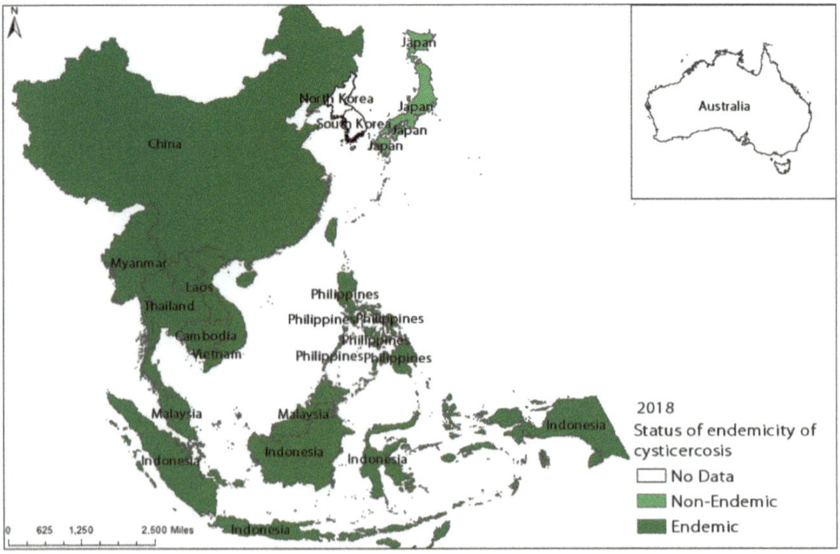

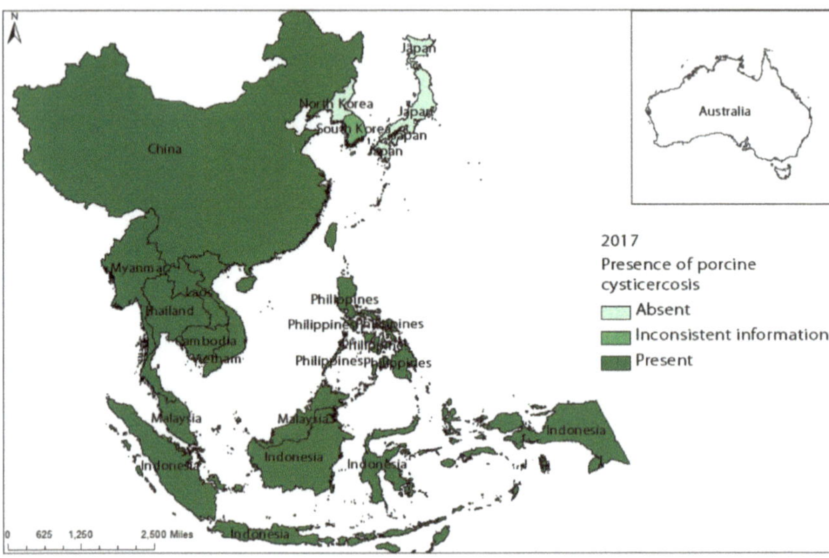

Only South Korea and Japan are not available to access the *Cysticercosis* data.

1.3 Foodborne trematode infections

Foodborne trematodiases are caused by trematode worms (flukes), among them the species affecting humans with potentially severe outcomes, are

Clonorchis, *Opisthorchis*, *Fasciola* and *Paragonimus*. *Clonorchiasis* and *opisthorchiasis* are confined to Asia, while *paragonimiasis* can be found in Africa, Asia, and Latin America. *Fascioliasis* is a global disease, affecting a significant number of countries throughout the world.

In this map we collect the data from WHO https://www.who.int/foodborne_trematode_infections/en/ by using the infection areas among 12 countries.

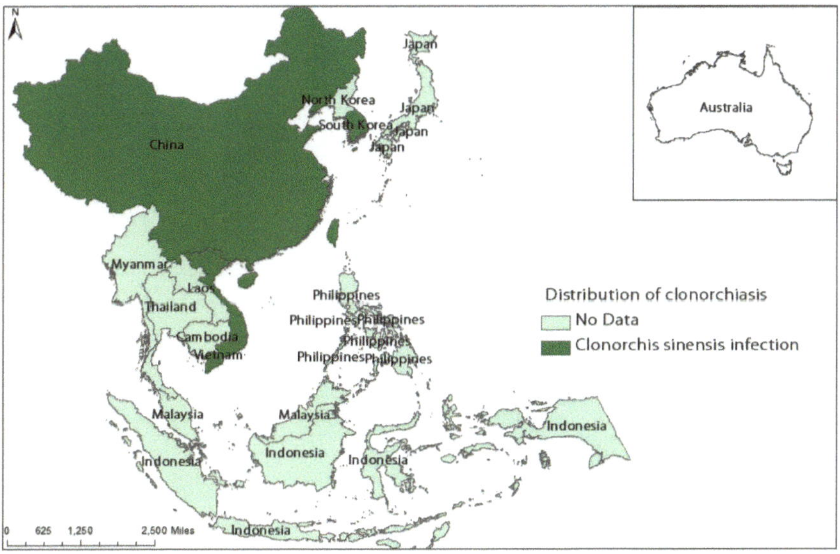

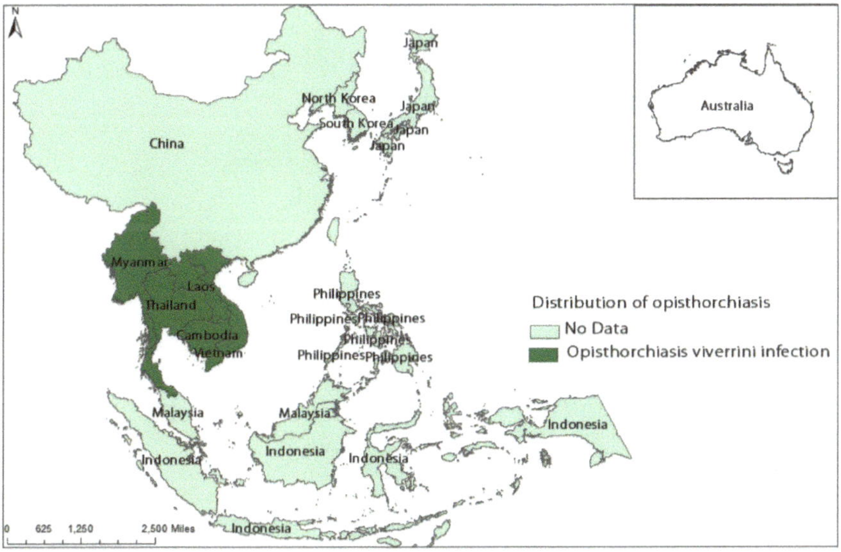

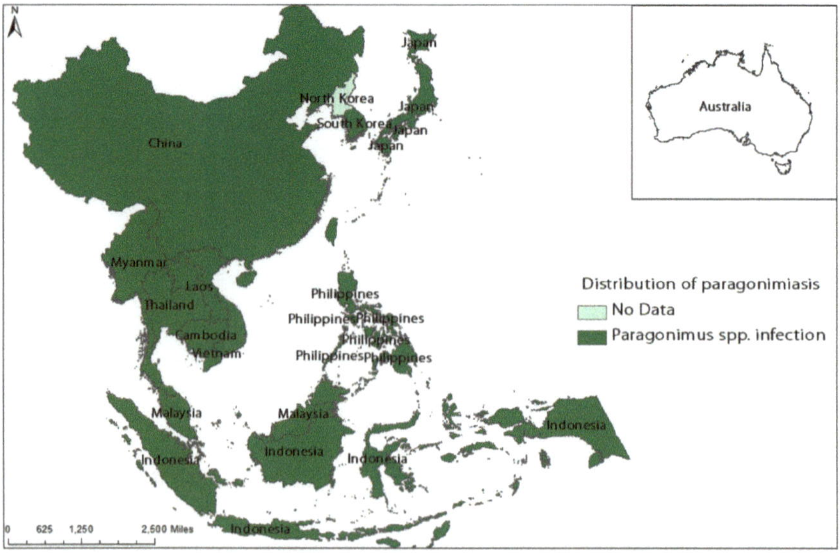

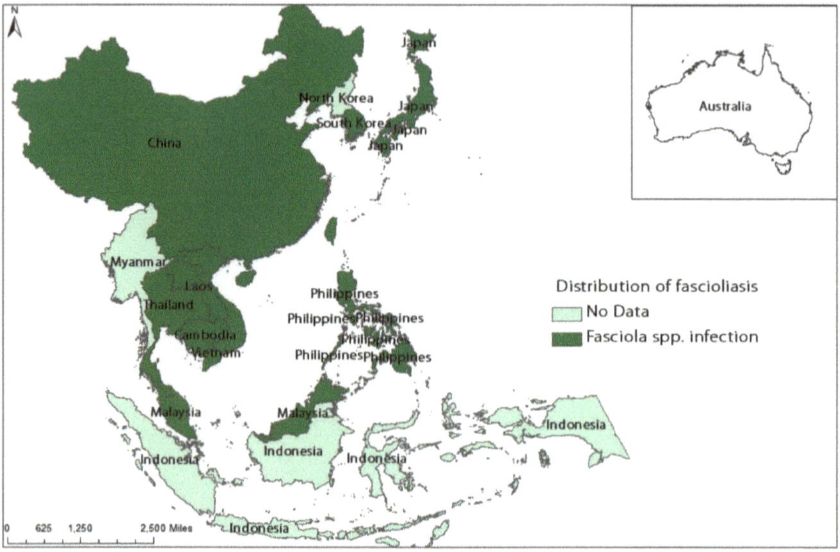

Countries in Asia are the worst affected.

2. Further reading

Food and Agriculture Organization of the United Nations, World Health Organization, 2014. Multicriteria-Based Ranking for Risk Management of Food-Borne Parasites.

Mutapi, F., Maizels, R., Fenwick, A., et al., 2016. Human schistosomiasis in the post mass drug administration era. Lancet Infect. Dis. 17 (2) e42–e48.

Taenia solium, 2019. WHO endemicity map update.

World Health Organization, 2013. WHO Estimates of the Global Burden of Foodborne Diseases.